Therapeutic Nursing

Improving Patient Care through Self-awareness and Reflection

EDITED BY DAWN FRESHWATER

SAGE Publications
London • Thousand Oaks • New Delhi

SAGE Publications Ltd
6 Bonhill Street
London EC2A 4PU

SAGE Publications Inc
2455 Teller Road
Thousand Oaks, California 91320

SAGE Publications India Pvt Ltd
32, M-Block Market
Greater Kailash - I
New Delhi 110 048

British Library Cataloguing in Publication data

A catalogue record for this book is available from
the British Library.

ISBN 0 7619 7063 0
ISBN 0 7619 7064 9 (pbk)

Library of Congress Control Number: 2001 135910

Typeset by C&M Digitals (P) Ltd., Chennai, India
Printed in Great Britain by TJ International Ltd, Padstow, Cornwall

Contents

List of Figures and Tables

Figures

Tables

List of Contributors

Jill Down is a Practice Development Nurse who has a vast amount of clinical expertise in the intensive care setting. She has set up and run a clinical supervision project within the unit and explored the use of herself as a therapeutic tool in the critical care environment.

Dawn Freshwater is Professor of Mental Health and Primary Care at Bournemouth University. She is currently leading the development of an academic research centre in mental health and primary care practice in North Dorset Primary Care Trust. Her research programme focuses on critical reflexivity, reflective practice and the development of practitioner-based research methods for practice improvement.

Roderick McKenzie is currently practicing as a Community Psychiatric Nurse specialising in addiction with the Highland Primary Care NHS Trust. Since qualifying as a nurse in 1992 he has been clinically based, with work experience encompassing the broad spectrum of psychiatric nursing care including; continuing care, rehabilitation, care of the elderly mentally ill and acute psychiatry.

Tessa Muncey is principal lecturer at Homerton College, School of Health Studies, Cambridge. Her time is divided between managing the Entry to Register (Nursing) programme and running a Masters degree in Primary and Community Care. The focus of her recent research has been teenage pregnancy and psychological profiles of student nurses.

Marilyn E. Parker is Professor of Nursing and founding Director of the Centre for Innovation in School and Community Well Being at Florida Atlantic University. The focus of her scholarship in recent years includes developing multidisciplinary integrated practice in communities of underserved immigrant populations in Palm Beach County, Florida.

Carol Picard is Associate Professor and Associate Director of the graduate Nursing Program at the MGH Institute of Health Professions in Boston, Massachusetts. Her program of research investigates the experience of illness and meaning of health for persons with chronic and life-threatening conditions.

Jacqueline Randle is Lecturer at the School of Nursing, University of Nottingham. Her chief interests are sociological perspectives of power relationships and transformatory educational practice.

Gary Rolfe is Reader in Practice Development Research, School of Health and Social Care, University of Portsmouth. He has a particular interest in action research, advanced practice and student-centred multi-disciplinary education. He teaches and facilitates research and practice development to health and social care practitioners from a wide range of professional backgrounds.

Gillian Todd is a currently a National Health Service Research Fellow studying for a PhD in Psychiatry at Cambridge University. She is a Registered Mental Health Nurse and worked as a Community Psychiatric Nurse for 15 years. She is also a practising Cognitive Psychotherapist.

A. Lynne Wagner is Professor of Nursing and Poetess, Department of Nursing, Fitchburg State University, Boston. Lynne, whose doctorate focused on Leadership in Schooling, is certified as a Lamaze Childbirth Educator and a Family Nurse Practitioner. She has had a private practice in childbirth education for 30 years and has worked in various nursing settings.

Preface

Nursing is an experience that occurs between two people; it is a deep experience that cannot always be adequately communicated to another person. Paradoxically, there is no doubt that the practice of nursing occurs within an interpersonal interaction, in the absence of which nursing becomes an empty routine. *Therapeutic Nursing* attempts to capture the atmosphere of the nurse–patient relationship, exploring not only the interpersonal but also the intrapersonal. These are inextricably linked as the individual's self-understanding is enormously enhanced by coming up against the personal understanding of another. Today, more than ever before, nursing is being constructed around the centrality of the nurse–patient relationship, which is conceived of as equal partnership and it is through the establishment of a therapeutic 'healing association' that nurses are said to promote healing (Allen, 2000: 184).

Recent efforts have also been made to change the nature of the patient–professional relationship by addressing the traditional power imbalance between service users and healthcare professionals (Allen, 2000: 183). Further, nurses are now encouraged to develop close relationships with patients so that they can understand the meaning their illness has for them and to use this knowledge to jointly plan individually tailored care. But what is the intended outcome of these nursing interventions and what is the most effective therapeutic tool that a nurse possesses in the execution of the plan of care?

These and other questions provided some of the initial momentum for the development of this book. Beginning with a simple but bold idea, namely that all nursing interventions are expressions of the personhood of the nurse, this text explores how the personhood of the nurse is used in creating an environment in which the therapeutic potential of both patient and nurse might flourish. Opportunities for learning answers to such questions, *with* the patient, exist in a wide variety of specialist healthcare settings, with practice providing a 'research space' within which we can study, amongst other things, the dynamic that is therapeutic nursing. Such praxis-oriented practice is based on the nurse–patient encounter as transformative and requires reflexive and reflective practitioners. Reflective practice provides space for healthcare providers to enter into a new dialogue and relationship with their patients, which helps begin the journey of healing. As such the concepts of reflective practice and critical reflexivity are guiding principles throughout the text, which is based on the premise that self-awareness and self-evaluation are prerequisites for autonomous, accountable, therapeutic nursing.

Drawing upon postmodern and post structural thought, *Therapeutic Nursing* offers an integrative, imaginative and applied perspective on the therapeutic use of self in nursing. I invite you to explore the role of therapeutic nursing whether your primary practice is nursing, teaching or researching. It is a book for all those willing to reflect on and develop themselves and their work. The broad focus of the book is reflected in the participating authors and the intended audience; authors are drawn from fields of mental health, primary care, acute care, nurse education, practice development and research. They are artists, poets, potters, dancers and musicians. The text is divided into three sections loosely based around therapeutic use of self as practitioner, educationalist and researcher. These, however, are not separate entities; what most obviously binds them is that they are all aspects of the therapeutic self. In this sense the book is representative of the many facets of the self, at any one time one facet may be more foreground than another and there are many more facets than this text can cover. But we do not pretend that this book can provide a whole picture, it is merely a partial view, one which aims to add to the ongoing conversation regarding therapeutic nursing in the hope that the conversation will be taken up by you, the reader. I invite you into the text in the hope that you will find some resonances with the questions, insights and ideas raised, and that this will stimulate further questioning about your own therapeutic practice.

Borrowing from Symington (1992), I suggest that the subject matter presented here is less important than the way it is treated. Thus if you are hoping to learn all that there is to know about therapeutic nursing, you will come away disappointed, for I believe, as Thomas Aquinas' intuited, that too much information blocks the act of understanding. Instead the text has embraced the Hebrew way. As Symington points out, 'The Hebrew way is to go round and round a subject, each time using different images to illuminate what is most profound' (1992: 11). Hence the intention is to convey the spirit of the therapeutic relationship and not the letter.

I would like to thank the many people who offered assistance and encouragement throughout the duration of this project. The staff at Sage have my appreciation for their efforts and in particular Alison Poyner, who provided encouragement at a very early stage and who was chiefly responsible for giving this project a chance. I would like to acknowledge the influence and inspiration of Professor Veronica Bishop. Finally, I would like to express my appreciation to the authors themselves for their creative and imaginative efforts.

Dawn Freshwater

References

Allen, D. (2000) 'I'll tell you what suits me best if you don't mind me saying: "lay participation" in health care'. *Nursing Inquiry*, 7: 2, 182–90.
Symington, N. (1992) *The Analytic Experience*. London: Free Association Books.

1 The Therapeutic Use of Self in Nursing

Dawn Freshwater

The nature and/or the existence of the 'self' is a topic that is well rehearsed in the literature surrounding healthcare. Indeed the notion of what constitutes the self is a subject that has interested poets, artists and philosophers alike. Writers have described theories of self in philosophical terms (Satre, 1956), theories of self in psychological terms (Laing, 1961; Freud, 1963; Lacan, 1966), in spiritual and transpersonal terms (Rowan, 2001; Wilber, 1981), in biological terms (Ginsburg, 1984), modernist terms (Giddens, 1990) and more recently postmodernist terms. Postmodern versions of the self challenge both the permanence and indeed the presence of a self at all, that is in the sense usually proposed (Fee, 2000; Flax, 1990; Gergen, 1991; 1997). Whilst definitions of the self derived from these varying theoretical perspectives are diverse, there is also some convergence. This chapter explores some of these definitions, reflecting upon the meaning of the self in the therapeutic alliance both for the nurse and the patient. Introducing the concepts of the self, self-awareness, self-efficacy, self-esteem and the therapeutic use of self, this introductory chapter aims to signpost the basic ideas under consideration within subsequent chapters.

Recent debates divide the theories of the self into two types, those of ego and bundle theories (Gallagher & Shear, 1999). Ego theories (in some way the most natural way to think about the self) believe in a persistent self. A self that is the subject of experiences and whose existence 'explains the sense of unity and continuity of experience' (Blackmore, 2001: 525). This equates with the dominant modernist viewpoint which will be outlined in more detail shortly. Bundle theories deny any such thing. As Blackmore points out, 'The apparent unity is just a collection of ever changing experiences tied together by such relationships as a physical body and a memory' (2001: 525). This perspective can be likened to the postmodernist perspective of the self which it would seem is becoming ever more inescapable.

The self

Consideration of the nature of the self is deeply bound up with questions about consciousness, about which the scope of this book does not allow an in-depth exploration. Hence whilst the fathomless abyss of consciousness and unconsciousness, reality and subjectivity are fundamental to any exploration regarding the nature of the self, the subsequent discussion will be limited to points of contextual relevance. In addition, there may be a number of contradictory standpoints presented simultaneously within this chapter; I do not apologise for this, rather I encourage the reader to tease out these inherent contradictions in the understanding that the self is in fact a contradictory being, if indeed a self does exist. The reader is encouraged to pursue further writings as indicated in order to expand the ongoing conversation pertaining to the nature of the self.

It has been argued that the concept of a self possessed by a person is a product of both personal reflection and social interaction. Priest's defines the self as 'an individual that is conscious of the individual that it is while at the same time being conscious that it is the individual it is conscious of' (1991:163). The experiencing self as described by Bohart (1993) and Maddi (1989) is essentially anti-reductionist in nature. Life is apprehended through experiencing, which involves an interplay of thought and feeling, without either of these concepts being conceived of as polar opposites (Bohart, 1993). Humanistic psychologists, however, describe the self as conceived of separate entities. Rogers (1991), for example, speaks of the organismic self and the self-concept. The organismic self is that aspect of the self which is essentially the 'real' inner life of the person and is present from birth. The organismic self consists of the basic force that regulates the individual's physiological and psychological growth; growth and maturity are seen as the central aims of this aspect of the self (Hough, 1994; Rogers, 1991). Therefore the focus of the organismic self is essentially internal. This view of the self purported by humanistic psychology has recently been challenged by social constructivism, deconstruction and postmodernism. All of these theories say in their own way that there is no 'real' self as defined in the sense usually proposed by humanistic and modernist theories.

As some authors have observed, the dominant modernist view specifies that the self is a 'finite, rational, self-motivated and predictable entity which displayed consistency with itself and across contexts and time' (Gottschalk, 2000: 21). Hence from a modernist perspective the self can be either healthy or pathological; it could also be observed, diagnosed and indeed improved. Postmodern theory, however, challenges this assumption, positing that the self is a conversational resource, that is to say, it is a story we tell to others and ourselves. Androutsopoulou, for example, states that from the narrative and social constructivist viewpoint the self:

> ... equals to a continuous construction of a self-narrative, aiming to secure a sense of historical continuity, directionality and coherence among what often appear to be loosely connected 'selves' that may seem to act differently depending on the circumstances. (2001: 282)

Thus the 'solid and stable modern self loses its' footing and becomes fluid, liminal and protean self*hood*' (Gottschalk, 2000: 21, original italics). Postmodern theories then move beyond the concept of a stable and static self, rendering it obsolete, to the notion of the self as a continuous process, constituted through multiple and often contradictory relationships. Thus the self as postmodern selfhood is iterative, interactive and interdependent. This has obvious implications in the context of a book which focuses on the therapeutic use of the self in work which is largely relationship based; namely that of nursing.

The self as a concept and self-concept

The very conception of a self is conceived of as a by-product of the relationship between power and knowledge; it is inseparable from language games, from mass media and ideologies, and as Gergen (2000) comments, loses its sense of substance in the ongoing construction and dissolution encountered within everyday relationships. He says of the self 'increasingly we find no "there" there' (2000: 100). Hence self-identity becomes a reflexively organised endeavour constructed through intrapersonal and interpersonal dialogue (Freshwater & Robertson, 2002). Nevertheless, there are a multitude of theories and an ever-increasing amount of literature being written concerning the self and its various aspects. One such aspect is that of the self-concept.

According to Burns the self-concept is 'forged out of the influences exerted on the individual from outside, particularly from people who are significant others' (1982: 9). This definition is in accord with the humanistic school of psychology, which views the self-concept as the individual's perception of himself, based on life experience and the way he sees himself reflected in the attitudes of others (Rogers, 1991).

According to this theory, the self-concept is acquired very early on in life and is continually reinforced by ongoing communications with significant others throughout life. As the self develops it needs to feel loved and accepted and as a result the organismic self (or the 'real' self) is neglected in favour of the self-concept. This is a point that Maslow (1970) illustrates in his hierarchy of needs (See Figure 1.1).

These ideas are not dissimilar to the theories of self developed by Carl Jung (1960). The self-concept can be likened to Jung's idea of the persona, with the psyche sitting closely to the organismic self. For Jung, the self was buried in the

Need for
Self-actualization
(Am I myself?)
Recognition needs
(Am I successful/repected?)
Belonging needs
(Am I loved, do I belong?
Safety Needs
(Am I safe/comfortable?)
Physiological needs
(Will I survive?)

Figure 1.1   *Maslow's hierarchy of human needs (1970)*

unconscious and full of creative potential. Jung believed that the aim of the psyche was towards individuation, that is the growth of an individual towards becoming aware of all aspects of their personality, leading to a better balance between their internal and external worlds and a subsequent integration of opposites. Through the process of socialisation, the self is repressed and thwarted; a persona (or mask) is developed as the individual becomes absorbed in enacting roles. Thus the individual becomes alienated from who they are and who they might become. Self-alienation, in this sense, meaning that in which the 'subject is no longer the author of the ongoing narrative of his self' (Dawson, 1998: 164), implying a loss of control over the self.

The focus of the self-concept is predominantly external. Rogers (1991) believed that the tendency of the organismic self was towards harmony and integration of discomfort arising as a result of inconsistency in ideas and feelings between the organismic self (the inner) and the self-concept (the outer). Burns (1982) contends that the self-concept has three roles, one of which is that of maintaining consistency, the other two being determining how experiences are interpreted and providing a set of expectancies. Where consistency is not maintained, a degree of dissonance is experienced (Festinger, 1957) and the discomfort that this causes is likely to motivate the individual to take action towards harmony and comfort, at any cost. It is often the awareness of discomfort with self that motivates the individual to engage in reflection. Such reflection, when undertaken in relation to nursing practice, often leads to the practitioner examining the contradictions between their espoused theories (desired practice) and their theories in action (actual practice) (Arygris and Schon, 1974).

Self-concept in nursing

The self is an important concept in nursing as in any therapeutic alliance, for often when patients are physically ill or psychologically distressed 'the most striking and consistent feature reported is a changed self-concept' (Dawson, 1998: 164). The goal of any therapeutic alliance (and incidentally emancipatory and transformatory learning, a topic that is considered in more detail in Part II of this book) is to facilitate the emergence of the authentic self (Friere 1972; Hall, 1986). In his recent work refining the humanistic approach to human inquiry, John Rowan (2001) writes of the authentic self (which he also refers to as the true self, the real self and the Centaur). The authentic self, he determines, lies beyond self-images, self-concepts and sub-personalities; requires that the individuals take responsibility for being themselves and for being 'fully human' (2001: 115). In this sense Rowan aligns the authentic self with the mystical self and draws heavily on the existentialist traditions and the work of Ken Wilber (1996; 1997). So, for Rowan and others the real or authentic self, when fully autonomous, can assume responsibility for being-in-the-world (Heidegger, 1972).

There is a Hasidic tale that illustrates Rowan's point beautifully:

Before his death, Rabbi Zusya said 'In the coming world, they will not ask me "Why were you not Moses?" They will ask me "Why were you not Zusya?"'

Rogers also captures the centrality of this point when reflecting on the work of Kierkegaard, whom he says:

... pictured the dilemma of the individual more than a century ago, with keen psychological insight. He points out that the most common despair is to be in despair at not choosing, or willing, to be one's self; but that the deepest form of despair is to choose to 'be another than himself'. On the other hand 'to will to be that self which one truly is, is indeed the opposite of despair', and this choice is the deepest responsibility of man. (1961: 110)

From this vantage point the role of the nurse in caring can be seen to be to transcend the self-concept, the persona (or what Winnicott (1971) might term the false self) in order to give voice to the organismic self, authentic self and to encourage, through a therapeutic alliance, the emergence of the authentic self of the patient (Rogers, 1991). This process necessitates a great deal of self-awareness and self-consciousness, a subject that will be touched on briefly in the following section. However, this is probably a good point at which to introduce some scepticism in relation to the idea of a self-concept and an organismic real self. As I mentioned at an earlier juncture, postmodern theories question the whole idea of a real self; from this particular stance there is no such thing as 'being authentic (true to oneself) or autonomous (taking charge of one's life) or self actualisation (being all that one has it in oneself to be), (Rowan, 2001: 120). Rowan, however, works hard to reinstate the real self in his latest work on action research and the reader is pointed to this for an interesting and in-depth analysis (and indeed defence) of the idea of a real self (Rowan, 2001). Discussions on the real self, self-concept and authentic self cannot take place in isolation from Freud's (1963) theories of the ego. In an earlier paper I attempted to highlight the impossibility of the human ego to perceive unity or wholeness, saying that 'Immediately I call myself "I", I cut myself off from everything that is "not I"'(Freshwater, 1999a: 136). Consciousness, splitting and dissecting experiences into pairs of opposites as it does, forces us to encounter the dualistic (and indeed pluralistic) nature of the self. It is to the idea of consciousness and the self that I now turn my attention, linking this to the theory of reflection and the notion of intentional action.

Self-consciousness and awareness of the 'I'

The practice of reflection is a central skill in developing an awareness of the self. The 'I' being self-conscious disappears in repetitive doing and is only found again when reflected upon (Spinelli, 1989). The process of repetition of routine tasks and focus on 'doing' (something that tends to dominate nursing, see Menzies, 1970) leads to a loss of 'I' or the self. Reflection on self is proposed as helping the practitioner to reform their identity through being in relation with themselves, the patient and others, instead of having an identity that is forged by their surroundings. Without reflection the practitioner may not be aware of the loss of self, which often manifests itself in somatic and psychological symptoms such as burn-out, disconnectedness and a sense of meaninglessness. Furthermore, practice, which is not reflected on either after the event or reflexively during the event, is not necessarily intentional practice.

According to Burks the concept of intentional action 'is especially relevant for those whose goal it is to change or maintain behaviour.' She goes on to say that 'In many nursing situations the intent of the nurse is to influence the action or behaviour of the client' (2001: 668). But not all action in nursing is intentional, in that it does not necessarily include mental processing neither of the intent nor of the conscious deliberative plan. This is to say that it does not always include an awareness of the (aspect of the) self that is practising. Bandura (1991) proposes that self-regulation and self-influence are the motivating factors in purposeful human action and whilst self-regulation is a multifaceted phenomenon, significant components of effective self-regulation include self-observation and monitoring of self-efficacy. Reflective practice provides such an opportunity for critically reflexive observations of self as practitioner and person, placing the self as central agent in the dynamic process of creative, autonomous and accountable practice. As Burks comments, 'intentional action originates from an actor's desires and wishes, it is influenced by motivation, emotional state, and the concept of self as the active agent' (2001: 669). Nursing theorist Peplau argued for ideas similar to this in 1952 when she asserted that 'Self insight operates as an essential tool and as a check in all nurse–patient relationships that are meant to be therapeutic' (1952: 12).

Knowing and recognising self through self-awareness and self-consciousness then can be seen to be fundamental to the development of a caring alliance which is to be therapeutic. As Boykin comments, 'The importance of knowing self as caring cannot be overemphasised as one can only understand in another what is understood in oneself' (1998: 44).

Self-recognition

Most human beings are born into a culture in which the mirror is a significant artefact (Miller, 1998). In such a culture the act of self-inspection is spontaneous and recurrent. But how do we succeed in recognising our own reflection if we do not know what we look like until we look in the mirror, how can we tell that the reflected face is ours? Miller posits that the individual 'in recognising everything else that appears in the mirror as a duplicate of what we can see around us, we might deduce the identity of our own reflection by a process of elimination since it would be the one item appearing in the mirror for which there were no counterpart in the immediate environment' (1998: 135). He goes on to comment that a much more significant clue regarding the identity of the image in the mirror is that 'its behaviour is perfectly synchronised with our own' (1998: 135).

But where is the optimum place for the development of self-awareness and even self-regard, for such needs are often linked to the negative attributes of vanity, self-absorption and narcissism. Narcissus, the most (in)famous example of an individual to be annihilated by reflective self-absorption, has been depicted as someone who fell in love with himself and as a result suffered a fatal outcome. But as Ovid asserts in *Metamorphoses,* Narcissus fell for his own self-reflection without recognising that he was looking at himself.

If psychotherapeutic practice and developmental theories are to be believed, then one of the most effective arenas for discovering the self is in a therapeutic relationship; that is, a relationship that facilitates such discovery in a safe and contained manner. Being with other people allows the individual to become aware of themselves through a variety of different experiences, including as Taylor (1998) suggests, through self-likeness. Self-likeness is when people see themselves mirrored in other people. Taylor advocates that in nursing 'self-likeness creates the potential for patients and nurses to understand the humanness of themselves on others, sharing an affinity as humans together bonded by the commonality of their ordinary human existence' (1998: 70).

Coming to know self as human through reflection is a complex and often confusing, if not demanding, call for nurses not least because pride, vanity and self-intoxication seem to come hard for those in the caring professions (as for other sectors of contemporary society), where it is not safe to speak of, let alone enjoy self-love (Watson, 1998). Much of the research examining self-esteem in nursing and the caring professions concludes that contextual factors conspire to diminish the self-esteem and subsequently the efficacy (and therapeutic potential) of the nurse resulting in self-doubting, submissive and often disillusioned practitioners (see for example Chapters 3, 5 and 9 in this book) (Freshwater, 2000).

Self-esteem, self-efficacy and self-regard

Self-esteem is commonly defined as the evaluative aspect of the self; it is a popular concept in the professional discourse surrounding the self and is often linked to the notion of self-regard. Whilst social psychologists usually relate self-esteem to the evaluative aspect of self-regard, other writers put forward self-esteem as a derivative of the affective dimension of the self, for example, whether one feels good or bad about oneself. It is also linked to self-knowledge, thus 'Reflexivity prompts an emotional response to self, and that is the fundamental reality to which self-esteem refers' (Hewitt et al., 2000: 170). Hewitt et al. endorse this association further stating that 'Self esteem (and its associated terms of reference) thus provides a label the person may attach to feelings aroused when he or she sees the self reflected in the social mirror' (2000: 171).

It appears that self-esteem resonates strongly in a culture that emphasises the centrality of the individual and that has a long tradition of discourse about the 'power of positive thinking' to help the person overcome obstacles, find success and enjoy happiness' (Hewitt et al., 2000: 171). Little wonder, then, that social theorists emphasise the connection between self-esteem and self-efficacy. Bandura (1986), for example, suggests that self-efficacy is related to levels and experience of self-confidence and self-concept, all of which are fundamental to the experience of self-esteem.

It is posited that is a 'good thing' for therapists, counsellors and healthcare workers, including nurses, to be self-aware in order to maximise their effectiveness when working with their clients (Bond & Holland, 1998; Boykin, 1998; Briant & Freshwater, 1998; Casement, 1985; Freshwater, 1998a; Higgs & Titchen, 2001). It has also been contested that in order to begin to understand and help other people, therapists, nurses and carers need to be aware of themselves. It is argued here that self-awareness does not only benefit relations with clients, but is crucial to the health and well being, and subsequently the self-esteem and therapeutic efficiency, of the practitioner.

There is much talk about the therapeutic use of self in the psychological literature (Casement, 1985; Sedgwick, 1994). As mentioned earlier, emphasis is placed on the necessity for the therapist to act with intention when acting in a therapeutic way, suggesting that a degree of self-awareness is required (Casement, 1985). As Jung (1960) proclaimed, 'the therapist must at all times keep watch over himself ... over the way he is reacting to his patients' (1960: 33). This is not to deny the therapeutic value of natural spontaneous emotional displays for clients, but one must have a 'self' available and be aware of that self in order to use it therapeutically.

Reflective practice is a way of viewing and participating in the unfolding drama of the self in becoming; the practitioner can watch themselves being invented as a therapeutic practitioner, engaging in intentional and deliberative practice, whilst at the same time be aware that they are inventing themselves. Hence 'Through the unfolding experience of reflection the nurse is looking backwards to the future, she is becoming whilst being', recognising his or her self as a dynamic and worthy being whose presence makes a difference (Freshwater, 1998b: 16). So, what has all this to do with therapeutic nursing and to return to a now familiar plea, what does it mean for the patient at the receiving end of the nursing (as if the practitioner is somehow not also the receiver)?

Therapeutic use of self

Originating in the field of psychotherapy, the concept of the therapeutic use of self is widespread throughout healthcare literature; little, however, has been documented regarding the experience of the therapeutic effect of nursing. Ersser (1998) points out that the concept of therapeutic use of self in nursing has been influenced by those nurse practitioners with a psychotherapeutic interest (see for example Peplau, 1952; Hall, 1969; and Travelbee, 1971).

As Ersser notes, and as alluded to previously in this chapter, emphasis is given to the importance of the nurse acting with intention when aiming to be therapeutic. Travelbee, for example, defines therapeutic use of self as 'When a nurse uses self therapeutically she consciously makes use of her personality and knowledge in order to effect a change in the ill person. This change is considered therapeutic when it alleviates the individual's stress' (1971: 19).

Ersser's (1997) own study challenges this notion, arguing that the therapeutic potential of the nurse's presentational actions may be 'communicated to the patient with or without intention' (1998: 56). Concluding that there is still a need to examine the nature of therapeutic nursing, Ersser calls for a re-examination of what he calls the 'received concept' of therapeutic use of self, one which allows for and values the nurses' 'natural, spontaneous emotional display for patients which is not intentionally purposeful' (1998: 56). One might question this call, for whilst some natural and spontaneous actions may not appear to be purposeful (see Winnicott's analysis of play, for example, 1971), there may still be intentionality which is not yet known. Other writers too, argue that all human action is undertaken to achieve a purpose or to execute an intention (Ewing & Smith, 2001; Langford, 1973). This is to say that 'all human actions, including nursing actions, reflect ideas, models, or some kind of theoretical notion of purpose and intention and how these purposes and intentions can be executed' (Freshwater, 1999b: 29). The exploration of these alternative vantage points form the beginnings of a response to Ersser's challenge to revisit the therapeutic use of self in nursing; this text provides a forum for debate regarding contemporary issues related to the concept of therapeutic use of self and indeed contemporary developments in therapeutic nursing in healthcare.

Therapeutic nursing?

McMahon (1998) identifies a number of characteristics that may affect the practitioner's ability to nurse therapeutically. Drawing on the work of Muetzel's (1988) models of activities and factors affecting the therapeutic nurse–patient relationship, McMahon validates the mutually beneficial relationship that is therapeutic nursing, emphasising the role of self-awareness and evaluation to achieve the same. Muetzel argues that the ability of the nurse to partake in a therapeutic relationship is dependent upon the nurse having developed as a person, both personally and professionally. Butler (1995) concurs, saying 'The qualities of the personal self within the professional are the key to excellence' and that 'professional development is radically centred in development of self' on 'personal being and becoming' and the 'understanding of individual human agency in the realm of practical actions' (1995: 153). Drawing upon Labone (1994), Ewing and Smith argue that 'In our development as practitioners we must continue to reconcile our ideal professional self and our actual professional self' (cited in

Higgs & Titchen, 2001: 25), indicating that the prevailing perception of a lack of integration with regards to the self, persists. This perhaps affirms the postmodern view that the self is not only fragmented but consists only of fragments tied together which can be integrated through the current self-narrative.

On the point of integration Field and Fitzgerald (1998) indicate the need for therapeutic nursing to be both integral to everyday practice, explicitly, in which it forms the foundation for all nursing, and discreetly, whereby specific therapeutic skills are practised within the context of a therapeutic alliance.

Self as worker – the professional self

It was suggested earlier that knowing self is a frequently unmet challenge by nurses, who usually have an inclination to focus on the behaviour and potentials of others finding it difficult to focus on them'selves'. Although paradoxically, it is the focus on other that very often brings self-appraisal; this is one of the rewards of doing the work. However, it has also been pointed out that the self (in modernist terms) develops a persona, a self-concept with which it faces the world. For some nursing authors this represents the schism between the professional self and the personal self, or what Taylor (1998) refers to as 'the ordinary self'. She suggests that:

> ...some nurses may choose to hide behind their professional masks and talk in high falsetto pitch to mimic the 'soapie' representations of a 'real' nurse. Acting out the role of a nurse may also serve to protect the hapless practitioner from the everyday battle-front of clinical work, where emotional knocks and bruises may be the norm.' (p. 74)

She goes on to say that in the uncertain context of professional practice 'a façade may act as armour to protect nurses from the daily drama of human suffering. In this sense, nurses are patients of sorts, in that they also suffer because of the illness experiences of the people for whom they care' (Taylor, 1998: 74).

So it would seem that, for the nurse, the professional self is defined in relation to others (namely patients) as it is for the client (namely the nurse). When discussing the self in relation to others, the word 'personality' is often used, and whilst it is not something that can be expanded upon here, it is important to note that the concept of a personality is of direct concern to this book (most notably Chapters 4, Part II and Chapter 9) in that it is closely linked to the issue of relationship.

The word 'personality' is used to describe the way people are perceived in relation to others. Their personality is the thing that distinguishes them from others. One might question if there are certain types of personality that are attracted to therapeutic work, or indeed does the personality attract the work? Perhaps, as Kolb explains, there is an interplay: 'Environments tend to change personal characteristics to fit them' (the process of socialisation perhaps linked to the earlier discussion regarding self-esteem and self-regard), however 'people tend to select themselves into environments that are constant with their personal characteristics' (1984: 143). What does seem important here is the level of self-awareness involved in making the decision to work with the selves of others and inherent in this decision is the level of conscious self-choice and perception of (internal) locus of control (as opposed to unconscious needs, perceived external locus of control) (Rotter, 1966).

The idea of a professional self is also directly linked to the theory of locus of control. As Rotter (1966) points out, work performance is closely aligned with the worker's locus of control; that is, whether nurses perceive outcomes as controlled by themselves or by external factors, this is obviously an important concept for practitioners when viewed in terms of the parallel processes with their patients, whom also will be negotiating power and control in the management of their health needs. Perception of control is important to the self and all individuals, whatever their walk of life. Rotter (1966) maintained that certain individuals believe that there is a strong link between what they do and what happens to them (originators of behaviour), while others deny or minimise this link and explain events on the basis of fate, luck or chance (non originators). Hence when individuals perceive the event to be dependent on their behaviour, they have an internal locus of control. If, on the other hand, they believe that they do not have any control over events and attribute success or failure to outside forces, they have an external locus of control. This also has implications for the patient who comes to the therapeutic alliance in search of some new learning which will re-instill in them a sense of self-control and self-reliance. Part I of this book provides examples of practitioners who are negotiating their way through the healthcare system, learning about themselves both as professionals and as powerful, self-determining human beings, originators of behaviour.

Self as learner – the developing self

Factors such as self-awareness and locus of control play a crucial part in the nurse and patient being open to new learning and expanding consciousness (and in turn self-awareness). As already revealed, Jung's (1971) opinion of the self mooted several different aspects to the personality, which strive to become integrated. He included in these, attitudes towards the outer world and ways of perceiving the world. Jung (1971) indicated four predominant ways of perceiving the world: thinking, feeling, intuition and sensing. In addition, individuals approach the world from either a predominantly extrovert or introvert manner. Although it should be noted that Jung maintained that a person's psyche contains all of these aspects, but in their development identify with a preferred way of translating information. Scales have been devised to measure the extent to which an individual has a preference for ways of relating to the world (Myers, 1980; Jung, 1971), Similarly, it is debated that individuals have a preferred style of learning (Kolb, 1984). It could therefore be argued that not only are different theoretical perspectives of the self required, but that the differing approaches to therapeutic use of self that are derived from the varying theoretical constructs are necessary in order to meet the diverse needs of the learning self.

These are significant considerations for the learning and teaching process as Field and Fitzgerald so poignantly articulate: 'The obvious corollary of therapeutic nursing is the development of practice-led curricula' (1998: 100), which concentrates upon the learner and 'the practitioner becoming responsible for and capable of controlling his or her own learning and practice' (1998: 101). Therefore, student-centred philosophies of education that include self-evaluation, student autonomy and education as life-long self-directed processes need to be fully embraced as part of the development of the therapeutic practitioner. Part II of this book outlines examples of student-centred philosophies that are not only firmly embedded within the nursing curricula, but are lived in everyday teaching practice in creative and therapeutic ways.

Self as researcher

It was posited earlier that the modernist conception of the self meant that it could be observed, diagnosed and improved. This rather objective language promotes a view of self-observation as if the self were being observed in an objectified manner by an (external) other, as opposed to a subjective investigation of oneself in dialogue and conversation with others (including oneself). For all the postmodern criticisms of humanistic psychology, it has promoted a view of research which involves treating research participants as human, and as was indicated earlier, humanness is deemed by some authors to be a fundamental component of therapeutic nursing (Taylor, 1998). As such the researcher is also human and does not hide behind roles; taking reflexivity seriously, the self as researcher does not exclude themselves from the research process, rather they see themselves as co-participants in the research endeavour.

This approach to research is not novel, although nursing still struggles to adapt to such radical perceptions of research in its drive towards evidence-based practice. What might be more novel is the idea that the process of the research itself might be therapeutic, that is to say, that the research itself is the therapy. Bentz and Shapiro (1998) applaud the contemporary development in therapeutic research stating that 'the contemporary situation in inquiry and research is one that is conducive to an integration of personal and philosophical self-reflection and also requires it' (p. 34). They go on to say that in their work with students 'we have observed over and over again the way in which the process of carrying out a research project seems to promote psychological and even spiritual development and transformation' (Bentz & Shapiro, 1998: 34).

This type of practitioner-based enquiry is called transformation because the people involved change; this includes all participants. But what makes reflexive inquiry transformational is the pattern of data collection, which is collaborative; in this sense the researcher is transformed from observer to participant. Engaging in reflexive research then means that all those involved are participants in the research endeavour, deconstructing the narratives that are created by and about self and about the therapeutic alliance. Part III of this book identifies ways in which practitioner-based research might transform and influence practice, and indeed self.

References

Androutsopoulou, A. (2001) 'Fiction as an aid to therapy: a narrative and family rationale for practice'. *Journal of Family Therapy*, **23**, 278–95.

Arygris, C. & Schon, D. (1974) *Theory in Practice Increasing Personal Effectiveness*. Massachusetts: Addison Wesley.

Bandura, A. (1991) 'Social Cognitive Theory of Self-Regulation'. *Organisational Behaviour and Human Decision Processes*, **50**, 248–87.

Bandura, A. (1986) *Social Foundations of Thought and Action: A Social Cognitive Theory*. New Jersey: Prentice Hall.

Bentz, V.M. & Shapiro, J.J. (1998) *Mindful Inquiry in Social Research*. California: Sage.

Blackmore, S. (2001) 'State of the Art: Consciousness'. *The Psychologist*, **14** (10), 522–5.

Bohart, A.C. (1993) 'Experiencing the basis of Psychotherapy'. *Journal of Psychotherapy Integration*, **3** (1), 51–67.

Bond, M. & Holland, S. (1998) *Skills of Clinical Supervision for Nurses*. Milton Keynes: Open University Press.

Boykin, A. (1998) 'Nursing as Caring through the Reflective Lens'. in Johns, C. & Freshwater, D. (eds) *Transforming Nursing through Reflective Practice*. Oxford: Blackwell Science.

Briant, S. & Freshwater, D. (1998) 'Exploring mutuality within the nurse–patient relationship'. *British Journal of Nursing*, **7** (4), 204–211.

Burks, K. (2001) 'Intentional Action'. *Journal of Advanced Nursing*, **34** (5), 668–75.

Burns, R. (1982) *Self Concept Development and Education*. London: Holt, Rinehart and Winston.

Butler, J. (1995) 'Designing for personal and professional excellence: The designer as lifelong learner' in Cachs, J., Ramsden, P. & Phillips, L. (eds) *The Experience of Quality in Higher Education*. Brisbane: Griffiths University, p. 153–74.

Casement, P. (1985) *On Learning from the patient*. New York: Guildford Press.

Dawson, P. (1998) 'The Self' in Edwards, S.D. *Philosophical Issues in Nursing*. London: Macmillan.

Ersser, S.J. (1998) 'The presentation of the nurse: a neglected dimension of therapeutic nurse-patient interaction?' in McMahon, R. & Pearson, A. (eds) *Nursing as Therapy*. Cheltenham: Stanley Thornes, Ch. 3.

Ersser, S.J. (1997) *Nursing as Therapeutic Activity: An ethnography*. Aldershot: Avebury.

Ewing, R. & Smith, D. (2001) 'Doing, Knowing, Being and Becoming: The nature of professional practice' in Higgs, J. & Titchen, A. (eds) *Professional Practice in Health, Education and the Creative Arts*. Oxford: Blackwell Science, Ch. 2.

Fee, D. (ed.) (2000) *Pathology and the Postmodern*. London: Sage.

Festinger, L. (1957) *A Theory of Cognitive Dissonance*. New York: Harper and Row.

Field, J. & Fitzgerald, M. (1998) 'Therapeutic Nursing: emerging imperatives for nursing curricula' in McMahon, R. & Pearson, A. (eds) *Nursing as Therapy*. Cheltenham: Stanley Thornes.

Flax, J. (1990) *Thinking Fragments*. Berkeley: New York University Press.

Freshwater, D. (1998a) *Transformatory Learning in Nurse Education*. Unpublished PhD Thesis. University of Nottingham.

Freshwater, D. (1998b) 'From Acorn to Oak Tree: A Neoplatonic Perspective of Reflection and Caring'. *The Australian Journal of Holistic Nursing*, **5** (2), 14–19.

Freshwater, D. (1999a) 'Polarity and Unity in Caring: The healing power of symptoms'. *Complementary Therapies in Nursing and Midwifery*, **5: 1**, 136–9.

Freshwater, D. (1999b) 'Communicating with Self through Caring: The student nurse's experience of reflective practice'. *International Journal of Human Caring*, **3** (3), 28–33.

Freshwater, D. (2000) 'Crosscurrents: Against Cultural Narration in Nursing'. *Journal of Advanced Nursing*, **32** (2), 481–4.

Freshwater, D. & Robertson, C. (2002) *Emotions and Needs*. Milton Keynes: Open University Press (in Press).

Freud, S. (1963) *Standard Edition of the Complete Psychological Works 1953–1974*. London: Hogarth Press.

Friere, P. (1972) *Pedagogy of the Oppressed*. Harmondsworth: Penguin.

Gallagher, S. & Shear, J. (eds) (1999) *Models of the Self*. Thorverton: Imprint Academic.

Gergen, K.J. (2000) 'Pathology and Selfhood: New and Contested Subjectivities' in Fee, D. (ed.) *Pathology and the Postmodern*. London: Sage, Ch. 5.

Gergen, K.J. (1997) 'The place of the Psyche in a constructed world'. *Theory and Psychology*. 7 (6), 723–46.

Gergen, K.J. (1991) *The Saturated Self: Dilemmas of identity in contemporary life*. New York: Basic Books.

Giddens, A. (1990) *The consequences of modernity*. Stanford: Stanford University Press.

Ginsburg, C. (1984) 'Towards a Somatic understanding of the self'. *Journal of Humanistic Psychology*, **24**, 66–92.

Gottschalk, S. (2000) 'Escape from Insanity: "Mental Disorder" in the Postmodern Moment' in Fee, D. (ed.) *Postmodern Pathology*. London: Sage. Ch. 2.

Hall, J.A. (1986) *The Jungian Experience*. Toronto: Inner City Books.

Hall, L. (1969) 'The Loeb Center for Nursing and Rehabilitation. Montefiore Hospital and Medical Center'. *International Journal of Nursing Studies*, **6**, 81–95.

Heidegger, M. (1972) *Being and Time*. New York: Harper and Row.

Hewitt, J.P., Fraser, M.R. & Berger, L. (2000) 'Is it me or is it Prozac? Antidepressants and the Construction of Self' in Fee, D. (ed.) *Pathology and the Postmodern*. London: Sage. Ch. 8.

Higgs, J. and Titchen, A. (2001) *Professional Practice in Health, Education and Creative Arts*. Oxford: Blackwell Science.

Hough, M. (1994) *A Pratical Approach to Counselling*. London: Pitman.

Jung, C. (1971) *Psychological Types*. Princeton: Princeton University Press.

Jung, C. (1960) *On the Nature of the Psyche*. Princeton: Princeton University Press.

Kolb, D.A. (1984) *Experiential learning: Experience as the source of learning and development*. New Jersey: Prentice Hall.

Labone, E. (1994) 'Teacher Burnout: Towards preventative strategies'. Paper presented at Australian Association for Research in Education Annual Conference, Newcastle, NSW. Nov.

Lacan, J. (1966) *Ecrits: A selection*. London: Tavistock.

Laing, R.D. (1961) *Self and Others*. New York: Pantheon.

Langford, G. (1973) *Human Action*. New York: Doubleday.

McMahon, R. (1998) 'Therapeutic nursing: theory, issues and practice' in McMahon, R. & Pearson, A. (eds) *Nursing as Therapy*. Cheltenham: Stanley Thornes.

Maddi, S. (1989) *Personality Theories: a comparative analysis*. Pacific Grove: Wadsworth.

Maslow, A. (1970) *Motivation and Personality*. New York: Harper and Row.

Menzies, I.E.P. (1970) *The Functioning of Social Systems as a Defence Against Anxiety*. London: Tavistock.

Miller, J. (1998) *On Reflection*. London: National Gallery.

Muetzel, P.A. (1988) 'Therapeutic Nursing' in Pearson, A. (ed.) *Primary Nursing in the Burford and Oxford Nursing Development Units*. Beckenham: Croom Helm.

Myers, I. (1980) *Myers-Briggs Type Indicator.* Palo Alto: Consulting Psychologists Press.

Peplau, H. (1952) *Interpersonal Relations in Nursing.* New York: Putnam.

Priest, S. (1991) *Theories of the Mind.* Boston: Houghton and Mifflin.

Rogers, C.R. (1991) *Client-Centred Therapy.* London: Constable.

Rogers, C.R. (1961) *On Becoming a Person.* Boston: Houghton.

Rotter, J.B. (1966) 'Generalised expectancies for internal versus external control of reinforcement'. *Psychological Monographs,* 80.

Rowan, J. (2001) 'The Humanistic Approach to Action Research' in Reason, P. & Bradbury, H. (eds) *Handbook of Action Research. Participative Inquiry in Practice.* London: Sage. Ch. 10.

Satre, J.P. (1956) *Being and Nothingness.* New York: Philosophical Library.

Sedgwick, D. (1994) *The Wounded Healer.* London: Routledge.

Spinelli, E. (1989) *The Interpreted World. An introduction to phenomenological psychology.* London: Sage.

Taylor, B. (1998) 'Ordinariness in Nursing as Therapy' in McMahon, R. & Pearson, A. (eds) *Nursing as Therapy.* Cheltenham: Stanley Thornes. Ch. 4.

Travelbee, J. (1971) *Interpersonal Aspects of Nursing,* 2nd edn. Philadelphia: F.A. Davis.

Watson, J. (1998) 'A meta-reflection on reflective practice and caring theory' in Johns, C. & Freshwater, D. (eds) *Transforming Nursing through Reflective Practice.* Oxford: Blackwell Science.

Wilber, K. (1997) 'An integral theory of consciousness'. *Journal of Consciousness Studies,* **4** (1), 71–92.

Wilber, K. (1996) *The Atman Project,* 2nd edn. Wheaton: Quest.

Wilber, K. (1981) *Up from Eden: A transpersonal view of human evolution.* London: Routledge.

Winnicott, D.W. (1971) *Therapeutic Consultations in Child Psychiatry.* London: Hogarth.

PART 1

THE PRACTITIONER'S PERSPECTIVE

Dawn Freshwater

This section begins with a chapter written by Roderick McKenzie who shares his experience of undertaking an autoethnographical research project. The development of therapeutic awareness though emerging self-knowledge and critical reflexivity as described by Roderick also sets the scene for subsequent chapters, which emphasise the significance of self-awareness in the therapeutic alliance.

Roderick, in conceptualising holism and writing of his chosen paradigm, reminds the reader of the dichotomies inherent in everyday practice, not least the theory–practice gap. Other nursing theorists have commented on the splits within nursing; American Theorist Margaret Newman, for example, referring to the dynamic tension between health and illness, points out that even placing seeming opposites on a continuum maintains the dichotomy. She argues that placing health and illness on a continuum:

> … maintains the dichotomy between the two by polarizing health at one end of the continuum and illness at the other end. If the goal of nursing is to move the individual toward health, then in this context, that means away from illness. In doing so, the dichotomy is maintained. (1994: 56)

Roderick also refers to the concept of holism, another value that has been widely discussed and accepted in nursing. As early as 1926, Smuts argued that the notion of therapeutic nursing was based on an underlying belief in holism which assumed that the mind and the body were inextricably linked. The literature that has evolved since Smuts' earlier propositions has a tendency to locate holism in opposition to fragmented care, paradoxically, in Newman's terms at least, perpetuating the dichotomy. One might question whether holism (as a concept) does anything to unify the splits within practice, or is indeed creating a further polarity in itself. If we were to problematise, as Ken Wilber (1982) does, the whole notion of holism, we could question whether there even is such a thing. As I discussed briefly in Chapter 1, the postmodernist theorists against holism query, from their sceptical viewpoint, the notion of a whole self. Perhaps, then, it is not so much nursing that is split, but the self that practices nursing. The splits experienced within everyday nursing practice are much more complex than they may at first seem. The postmodern paradigm views such dichotomies, and the contradictions which inevitably arise out of them, as forming part of the multi-layered context of reality and therefore of the self.

In discussing the concept of a paradigm, Roderick draws upon the writing of William Cody (2000) who speaks of the notion of borrowed theories. This is similar to the concept of received wisdom as posited by Belenky et al. (1986) in that the (often) passive process of accumulating facts and information about professional practice soon becomes the active process of using received wisdom as if it were the (my) truth. In this sense the practitioner actively chooses to be the passive recipient of received knowledge as opposed to having constructed their own practice wisdom, which demands an active processual relationship with the self. The view of self put forward by Roderick is that of a self that is co-created in relationship, a self that is simultaneously inventing itself whilst in the process of being invented. Thus the self as therapeutic practitioner is a dynamic and evolving entity whose theories, philosophies, beliefs and practices are constantly in the process of becoming (Parse, 1987).

This chapter challenges theorists to make explicit their underpinning paradigm and philosophy; but nurses, as applied theorists (and indeed applied philosophers), also need to make their theories explicit. For it is in so doing that they may become aware of the dichotomies and contradictions which serve as their guiding fictions. I use the term 'fiction' here, intentionally; the notion of narrative, story and fiction is something that is introduced early on in this book and is returned to repeatedly throughout. In this section in particular, both Roderick and Jill Downs make explicit reference to the significance of storytelling and narrative in the maturation of the therapeutic self. A growing number of practitioner/researchers from a variety disciplines have either taken the narrative turn or are in the process of 'converting'. That is to say that they are seeing individuals as organising their experience in the form of stories (Androutsopoulou, 2001). However, the rush to embrace narrative as a form of structuring the practice/research experience belies the amount of underlying confusion regarding the concepts themselves. In the literature the terms 'narrative' and 'story' get used interchangeably, with little exploration of the difference. Further, in the haste to appropriate narrativity as a research method in nursing and healthcare, one very important function of storytelling has been overlooked, that of the simple therapeutic value of telling the story itself and more importantly, of having it witnessed by an audience (Freshwater, 2001; Frank, 2000).

Epston et al. point out that whilst bibliotherapy (the private act of reading self-help and psychology books) is assumed to help the individual acquire skills and coping mechanisms to manage problems, they lack the presence of a 'legitimate audience' (1992: 109). But what constitutes a legitimate audience; doesn't oneself count as a legitimate audience? Another way of framing this question might be: does reflection require the presence of another (external) person? Such questions are crucial when viewed in the context of an autoethnographical case study or a reflexive action research study. What, for example, are the ethical considerations in undertaking critical reflexive research that places the self at the centre of the research process? How does one take care of the participant when the participant is oneself? Does caring for oneself require the presence of an (other)?

These questions may be worthy of further consideration, but I believe they should be approached with caution. For when the subjective is put under the microscope and macroscope, as it is in critical reflection, it runs the risk of becoming an 'it' as opposed to an 'I'. Perhaps, then, we need to be aware that in our eagerness to rescue subjective experience from the world of technical rationality, the approaches we choose, such as autoethnography and narrativity, hold the potential to become technical tools which in themselves submerse and subvert the subjective.

Jill Down picks up the discussion around caring as she explores the relationship between caring and nursing, providing an example of therapeutic nursing in a technological environment from the perspective of the critical care practitioner. There are many benefits of utilising technology in caring and nursing practices, but as Higgs (2001) notes, it has the potential both to serve and to depersonalise knowledge and practice. It is this process of depersonalisation, and of achieving the balance between instrumental and expressive skills to provide therapeutic nursing in a technologically caring situation, that is the focus of Jill's chapter. Jill, conceiving of the self within a phenomenological framework, uses John's (1998) philosophical framing to help answer the question 'How can the nurse be patient-centred when the response to the patient is one of mixed emotions and despair?

In the story of her work with Jenny, Jill writes of the difficulty of being therapeutic in extreme situations. The conception of nursing as therapy originated with the work of Lydia Hall (1963; 1964) who, rather than concentrate on the psychosocial aspects of nursing care, celebrated the physical. Thus Hall proposed that the central feature of therapeutic nursing practice was intimate physical touch. Jill, struggling to find a way through to connect to the person that is Jenny, rediscovers touch, signifying that technology is a tool, 'not an end in itself' (Higgs, 2001: 123).

Through the process of critical reflection, Jill journeys back to the heart of her caring beliefs as she revives her authoritative voice and her therapeutic potential. She grapples with the repersonalisation of her practice, expressing her concern and deliberations as she recounts the story of her encounter with Jenny. What is also noticeable in this, at times shocking, tale, is the challenge to be in the I–Thou relationship with the patient (despite all the machinery) as opposed to the I–It (Buber, 1958). Again references to the work of Buber and the I–Thou/I–It dichotomy will be found throughout the text; here it is particularly interesting to examine these ideas in relation to the implied power dynamics and the skill of patient advocacy. How easy is it for the practitioner to speak for or on behalf of the patient in situations where they struggle to find their own voice? The therapeutic role does include the skill of advocacy, particularly in the nurse–doctor–patient relationship, and whilst this may not be easy, the act of advocacy provides the practitioner with an opportunity to deconstruct the explicit and implicit hierarchical relationships within the therapeutic arena.

The struggle that Jill relates, to give voice to her embedded ethics of care, is not uncommon. Higgs, in discussing this, raises the question of whether or not nursing is going to partake in what he calls a 'culture of silence' (2001: 122) or engage in a more holistic and people-centred approach. Drawing on Friere's (1970) work on Socratic dialogue, he points out that no matter how submerged in a culture of silence, the individual practitioner is capable of critically examining the world through dialogue with others. Hence what Jill's chapter illustrates more than anything else is that therapeutic nursing requires a willingness to confront oneself and as such therapeutic nursing involves not only a high level of self-awareness and critical consciousness, but also an ongoing dialogue between the intrapersonal and the interpersonal.

This dynamic dialogic tension is the focus of Gillian Todd's chapter, which explores the internal dynamics of the developing practitioner. Drawing upon the work of Patrick Casement (1985) and using critical reflexivity, Gillian maps her progress as a clinical supervisor from reflection on action to reflection in action. Using a cognitive behavioural construct of the self, Gillian draws some useful parallels between the therapeutic alliance of the nurse and patient with that of the practitioner and supervisor.

Gillian's chapter examines how cognitive distortions may act as a barrier to accurate reflexivity; one such distortion is that such distortions exist, that is to say that within a cognitive behavioural context such distortions do exist, but perhaps the cognitive behavioural viewpoint is itself a distortion. Gillian bravely and creatively points out the parallels between Mezirow's (1981) levels of reflexivity and Beck et al.'s (1979) Cognitive Model. Brave, given the potential criticisms that might be levelled from a methodological standpoint regarding incongruencies of approaches. But to criticise this is to miss the point of the chapter, the development of the practitioner, who develops a personal theory of the processes involved in developing an internal supervisor and the subsequent effect of this on self-concept and clinical competence.

Whilst all three chapters present a differing perspective of the self and of the self as practitioner, what they all have in common is the notion of moving from received wisdom, or what Roderick refers to in his chapter as borrowed theories, to constructed wisdom. This is illustrated by both Jill and Gillian, who use the metaphor of finding of a voice. But it is not just the voice that is being constructed through critical reflection; it is also the therapeutic self as practice and practitioner become aware of intentional action.

References

Androutsopoulou, A. (2001) 'Fiction as an aid to therapy: a narrative and family rationale for practice'. *Journal of Family Therapy*, **23**, 278–95.

Beck, A.T., Rush, J.A., Shaw, B.F. & Emery, G. (1979) *Cognitive Therapy of Depression*. New York: Guildford Press.

Belenky, M.F., Clinchy, B.M., Goldberger, M.R. & Tarule, J.M. (1986) *Women's ways of knowing*. New York: Basic Books.

Buber, M. (1958) *I and Thou*. Edinburgh: T. and T. Clark.

Casement, P. (1985) *On Learning from the Patient*. New York: Guildford Press.

Cody, W.K. (2000) 'Paradigm Shift or Paradigm Drift? A meditation on commitment and trans-cendence'. *Nursing Science Quarterly,* **13** (2), 93–102.

Epston, D., White, M. & Murray, K. (1992) 'A proposal for re-authoring therapy: Rose's revisioning of her life and a commentary' in McNamee, S. & Gergen, K.J. (eds) *Therapy as a Social Construction*. London: Sage, 96–115.

Frank, A.W. (2000) 'The Standpoint of Storyteller'. *Qualitative Health Research,* **10** (28), 354–65.

Freshwater, D. (2001) 'Losing the Plot'. Paper presented at Texts, Narratives and Poetics Symposium. City University: London.

Friere, P. (1970) *Pedagogy of the Oppressed*. New York: Continuum.

Hall, L. (1963) 'A Centre for Nursing'. *Nursing Outlook,* **11,** 805.

Hall, L. (1964) 'Project Report. The Solomon and Betty Loeb Center at Montefiore Hospital and Medical Center, Bronx, New York'. *International Journal of Nursing Studies,* **6,** 81–95.

Higgs, C. (2001) 'Technology and the Depersonalisation of Knowledge and Practice' in Higgs, J. & Titchen, A. (2001) *Professional Practice in Health, Education and the Creative Arts*. Oxford: Blackwell Science.

Johns, C. (1998) 'Opening the doors of perception' in Johns, C. & Freshwater, D. (eds) *Transforming Nursing through Reflective Practice*. Oxford: Blackwell Science.

Mezirow, J. (1981) 'A critical theory of adult learning and education'. *Adult Education,* **32** (1), 3–24.

Newman, M. (1994) *Health as Expanding Consciousness*. St Louis: Mosby.

Parse, R.R. (1987) *Nursing Science: Major paradigms, theories and critiques*. Philadelphia: Saunders.

Smuts, J.C. (1926) *Holism and Evolution*. New York: MacMillan.

Wilbur, K. (1982) *The Holographic Paradigm and Other Paradoxes*. Boulder: Shambhala.

2   The Importance of Philosophical Congruence for Therapeutic Use of Self in Practice

Roderick McKenzie

When we stop inventing reality, then we see things as they really are.

Okri (1997)

Therapeutic use of self pertains to a particular collection of personal or human qualities consciously or deliberately employed when engaging with individuals in a therapeutic encounter, most commonly a counselling relationship but conceivably any helping or caring moment. Central to therapeutic use of self is the notion of self-awareness. However, we must also and by necessity consider the arena in which these qualities or skills are brought into play, that is the interaction between nurse and patient and the context within which this takes place. Assumptions that this encounter is a value-free encounter will be challenged within this chapter as I argue that therapeutic nursing takes place in a historical arena infused with competing paradigms including personal, professional and institutional codes and values. It is my intention to explore these issues with particular attention being paid to nursing's alliance with holism before providing examples of methods I have used in the pursuit of being self-aware.

Paradigms

The mere mention of the word 'paradigm' will have most folks scrambling for some metaphorical off button, but don't hit that button just yet! It is not surprising that many practitioners find the discussion surrounding differing paradigms challenging, if not confusing; the literature available related to the paradigm of research, knowledge and practice is multifarious, ambiguous and bewildering. I suspect that most practitioners find it hard to get turned on to such a debate and either wittingly or unwittingly switch off. Beyond this, discussions concerning paradigms are often crudely polarised, for example, the art/science, caring/curing debates in nursing and quantitative/qualitative debate in research. Crude because analysis of paradigms reveals that they are multi-layered and complex and this is seldom revealed in such discussions.

Mitchell and Cody (1993) assert that all theories flow from some philosophical paradigm or worldview. This is a vital point because it is rare that authors/ theorists make explicit the philosophy (and by association, paradigm) that under-pins their writing and theory. More often the philosophical roots are vague. Consequently, amid pressure to implement evidence or research-based practice the philosophy is lost and the theory–practice gap grows ever wider as practi-tioners struggle to understand why their practice does not 'feel' right.

Arguably, the most significant feature of nursing and nursing practice is that it sits within and is influenced by competing paradigms. Indeed, I would argue that the evolution of nursing is so inextricably linked with paradigms that it demands attention, and so in attending to this matter I will first of all examine the defini-tions of the elusive concept: a paradigm.

A paradigm is essentially a worldview specifying the basic assumptions and beliefs about the nature of reality (Kuhn, 1970). Powers and Knapp (1990) caution that the term 'paradigm' is sometimes used interchangeably with the term 'model'. A paradigm consists of a larger organising framework that contains:

1 Concepts, theories, assumptions, beliefs, values and principles that form a way for a discipline to interpret the subject matter with which it is concerned;
2 Research methods considered to be best suited to generating knowledge within this frame of reference;
3 What is open to investigation – priorities and views on knowledge deficit areas where research and theory building is most needed.
4 What is closed to inquiry for a time.

From this viewpoint, then, it can be seen that paradigms can be both exclusive and excluding; there may be flexibility *within* paradigms but not necessarily *between* paradigms. In nursing, the traditional scientific medical model has been the *ruling* or *dominant* paradigm for many decades; this is especially true of nursing research (Haggman-Laitila, 1997; Hopps, 1994; Fee, 2000; Watson, 1999). Hence it has been argued that nursing has inherited a legacy of positivism which promotes objectivity and reductionism while excluding subjective meaning and the personal (Playle, 1995). Paradoxically, given the dominance and influence of the ruling paradigm, it remains strangely invisible to nurses. This may be due to the fact that, as Kuhn (1970) observes, at any given point in the ongoing progress of a science, there is likely to be one dominant paradigm that is known as normal science. The convictions of this paradigm are taken by professionals as facts and taught as facts.

The paradigm shift

Fortunately, in my opinion, another feature of paradigms is that they are far from static; there will be movements or *shifts* within paradigms and from one paradigm to another. A paradigm shift in nursing is reflected in the ongoing development of nursing science. According to Cody (2000), nursing science has evolved through three distinct stages, these being:

1   The use of borrowed theories.
2   The use of use of theories specific to nursing, commensurate with the received view.
3   The use of theories specific to nursing *and challenging the received view* [emphasis in the original].

These stages and evidence of a paradigm shift are encapsulated within nursing education and by extension nursing practice. For example, as regards Cody's first and second stages, according to Apple (1988), textbooks as cultural commodities of our society often dictate what is legitimate knowledge. Fundamentally, the language of the core texts contained within the nursing curriculum shapes our views as nurses in training. A study in the US revealed that the meaning of nursing practice in core nursing textbooks was unquestionably determined by rationality and language that strongly favoured the view of nursing as a technical approach (Hiraki, 1992). Clearly this is consistent with the dominant paradigm.

Cody's third stage represents the paradigm shift, evidence for which, as mentioned, is considered to exist in nursing. For example, Johnson's (1990) bibliometric study analysis of nursing literature since 1966 depicts a shift from a traditional scientific model to a model based on holism. Sarter's (1988) analysis of four contemporary nursing theories reveals commonly shared themes, emphasising holism, process and self-transcendence and she suggests that it represents an emerging paradigm. Finally, Playle (1995) informs us that nursing and nurse education have been influenced by a shift towards a broadly humanist philosophy as a basis for practice.

As can be seen from the chronology of the citations, paradigm shifts are evolutionary and take time; however, a cautionary note is needed here, as I am not suggesting that some day the shift will reach a destination and stop, for the reality is that *constant evolutionary change is the only reality*. It is for this reason that an appreciation of paradigms and their effect is essential, for it is knowing where *you* are as the paradigm shifts that will be most important for your own practice and for the discipline of nursing.

To sum up, disciplinary knowledge progresses through aligning with or being influenced by a particular paradigm. This is perhaps one of the central problems within nursing, for as an emerging profession nursing has been attempting to establish its own unique body of knowledge and in this, two main issues emerge. Firstly, it is clear that nursing has never had a unique disciplinary vision; there has never been universal agreement on what the proper focus of nursing is or should be. Secondly, nursing has attempted to create its own unique body of knowledge by borrowing research methods and theories from other disciplines and in particular the natural sciences (Cody, 2000; Freshwater & Rolfe, 2001; Picard, 2000). So, while I have argued that the positivist, traditional scientific medical model remains the *dominant* paradigm in nursing research, education, and practice, nursing is in the midst of a paradigm shift.

Holism, nursings emerging dominant paradigm?

Horsefall (1995) believes that the scientific method is antithetical to the nursing values of holism. This view establishes holism as being in opposition to the dominant paradigm, for it is consistent with the tendency to polarise; we now know that it is not reductionism. Holism is emerging as an ideological construct with which we 'define' our disciplinary separateness. Given the breadth, depth and variety of writing on the subject, this is a position that nursing has clearly embraced. Significantly, as Seedhouse (2000) observes, all nurse theorists are in favour of holism in one form or another and there appear to be no papers by nurse academics against holism, although there is debate about what constitutes holism (Freshwater & Johns, 2001).

In brief, holistic nursing care approaches the patient as a whole. The individual is viewed as a biopsychosocial being having physiological, psychological, social and spiritual needs. Crucially, there is considered to be unity of mind, body and spirit (Oldnall, 1996; Pullen et al., 1996). Holism, then, holds that treatment must involve all of these factors. Furthermore, holism is both a philosophy and a practice/treatment modality. The key point that I wish to establish here is that for the discipline of nursing to progress, for the science to develop, nursing practice must be consistent with nursing philosophy and vice versa. Holism appears to be emerging as the key element within the evolving paradigm and in this, both defines the agenda and provides the means by which this position may be advanced. Finally, it is felt that holism represents a broadening of perspective on nursing's emphasis on a whole-person orientation that in turn stems from its tradition as humanistic practice (Kolcaba, 1997) and in this offers security, consistency and continuity of ideas and values. Central to these values must be honouring the primacy of experience and the subjective reality of our patients in providing individualised care. It is to this issue that I will now turn the attention of the reader, specifically exploring the concept of holism, therapeutic nursing and the effect of the dominant paradigm within mental health nursing.

Practicing and preaching

The activity of mental health nursing has several forms and takes place in many settings with different groups and individuals. Mental health nurses working in acute psychiatry, care of the elderly mentally ill, community psychiatric nursing, rehabilitation, family psychiatry, various specific 'therapist' groups and others, would all lay claim to their own particular character and identity. Mental Health Care in general is thought of as being a 'low-tech' branch of the nursing profession, but this is to ignore the counselling technologies; to refer back to my introduction, therapeutic use of self is most commonly associated with counselling and counselling lies at the centre of the vast majority of mental health work.

'Cognitivism' is a collective term for cognitive psychology and according to Rose (1994) represents the 'scientific' ground on which the counselling culture is camped. Cognitivism currently dominates Western psychology employing a computational metaphor for mental life that treats the operation of the mind as a form of internal computation representing the external world (Pickering, 1997). One of the problems with cognitivism is that it views experience and reality as at worst 'things' and at best isolated events, seldom or never as processes intimately enfolded in all of the aspects of an individual life as lived. To look at mental life as if it could be separated from the situation and from the form of life which gives it meaning is a reductive mistake (Pickering, 1997). Building on this philosophical position, Rose (1994) suggests that within counselling there is 'a technology of voices, a way of eliciting confession and responding to it through sequences of words and gestures often formulaic and specific to certain systems. To speak in the therapeutic encounter is to place ones words within a whole scientific field.'

In essence, then, the 'therapist' who restricts descriptions of experience to those phenomena that can be understood in terms of a known theory or diagnosis so that he can say something intelligible about them, leads to the problem of reduction, and in this reduces the individual to the status of object. We do this via signs, symptoms, diagnosis, models and exclusive language. This is a feature of what Cowling (2000) refers to as the 'clinicalisation' of human experience. Cowling is clear that clinicalisation is expressed in empirical, conceptual and theoretical approaches that miss the essential wholeness, variety and uniqueness of human existence. Models and theories impose order and rationality upon experiences and worlds that are in reality ambiguous, chaotic and problematic. This is not only contrary to holistic ideals, but also to nursing's commitment to caring for the 'whole person'. Despite the rhetoric of humanism and holism, it seems that nursing continues to objectify the patient.

Towards holism

The root of the objectification problem finds expression in Karl Jaspers' (1948) belief that the surrender of man's thinking to rationalism and of his artifice to technics have consequences that make him think that he is progressing, but make him neglect or deny the fundamental forces of his inner life. In surrounding ourselves with increasingly sophisticated theories and models we create the illusion of progress. In denying the primacy of experience by it's reframing within the counselling culture to match the theories and models, there is a very real or serious danger of alienating our patients.

Regarding the patient as a whole requires nothing less than the nurse acting as a whole person. The nurse who withholds parts of the self is unlikely to allow the patient to emerge as a whole person. And yet, nurses are expected to leave their own 'life' at the door on the way into work. As Sally Gadow (1993) says, the view that there is a separate 'nurse self' aligns with the traditional values that tend to view nurse as professional – a position that discourages the nurse from becoming personally involved. Ordinary human qualities are replaced with skills to be attained within the counselling technologies – ordinary human qualities such as empathy. But within a technology, empathy does not mean authenticity and contact does not mean connection. The only hope for the patient to be cared for in a holistic fashion lies with the ability of the nurse to be ordinary. Holism does not involve adding things on to the patient – signs, symptoms, labels and so on. To be truly connected one must instead strip away towards ordinariness.

As Taylor (1992) comments, the concept of person in nursing can take on a different meaning if nurses as humans are encouraged to see patients and nurses in terms of their oneness, rather than by their separateness. This echoes a principle that lies at the heart of Teilhard's (1959) vision, though it is rarely brought to the centre of his expositions, the principle that 'union differentiates'. This means that when two things unite to form one thing, or more correctly to form one community, then each by this union and communion becomes more full and different itself. Hence in keeping with Taylor's work, if I come to patient as nurse they become more fully patient. If I come to patient as person or 'self', then there is opportunity for them to become more fully person or self. So, ordinariness married to self-awareness is a crucial issue in nursing.

I would contend that if we are to practice holism, to approach the patient as a whole person in our own right, then we simply must have developed and be in tune with our own values. It should be a goal, if not ideal, of philosophically congruent holistic nursing that the values you practice by should be the ones which give meaning and sense-making to your own life. This, however, requires that the theory–practice gap be addressed and that theories in use are examined and articulated, a concern that has preoccupied many authors to date (see, for example, Freshwater & Rolfe, 2001; Freshwater, 1998; Rolfe, 1998; 1996; and further chapters in the current text).

The theory–practice gap

There is widespread acceptance that a theory–practice gap exists in nursing (Carr 1996; Hewison & Wildman 1996; Rolfe, 1998; 1996; Rolfe et al., 2001). Vaughan (1987) asserts that while practice and theory remain separate in nursing, students will experience a disparity between theory and practice. This in essence summarises the theory–practice gap; educators and researchers are seldom found in the environment of practising nurses. My argument, while acknowledging this, goes further in asserting that practice, theory and education have to be philosophically congruent. Counselling theories are well grounded in practice but, as I have argued, are often incongruous with the ideals of holism.

Parse (2001) appeals for nurses to be educated in the language of the discipline, arguing that every discipline has its own language. In supporting this principle I am also aware that the education of nurses still involves the importing of theories, and thus the language, of other disciplines, for example medicine, sociology, psychology and anthropology. Nurses are in effect speaking in tongues, a core feature of the theory–practice gap. One of the contemporary developments in nursing, that of reflective practice, appears to have the potential to resolve the theory–practice gap and promote philosophically congruent nursing.

Reflective practice

There has been growing interest in the development of reflective practice in the nursing profession, indeed Barton (2000) believes that reflection and reflective practice are terms that are very familiar to nurses and have become a feature of contemporary nursing practice. Reflective practice has been presented in the literature as something of a panacea with the potential to articulate knowledge locked in practice, promote freedom and growth for practising nurses and resolve the theory–practice gap. Most encouraging is the position that it is based on the personal foundation of experience. However, much of this acceptance, until recently, has been uncritical and in the pursuit of philosophical rigour I will, in the first instance, offer a brief critical review (Rolfe et al., 2001; Heath & Freshwater, 2000).

Within reflective practice there appears to be the tools to construct and view both ourselves and our practice within our wholeness, for example portfolio building, narrative, journaling and reflection, but, invariably it seems, the gaze is turned outward to the patient or used by others to construct the nurse by means of vignettes and so on. While the aim, in keeping with reflective practice, of vignettes, exemplars and narratives is to illustrate, illuminate and articulate theories in use, there are a number of methodological, philosophical and ethical dilemmas (Heath & Freshwater, 2000), so much so that one must seriously consider whether or not we should accept as valid all that is claimed on its behalf.

Methodological, philosophical and ethical dilemmas

Donald Schön (1983; 1987) has made a major contribution to the literature in describing the importance of reflection and is credited with having introduced the concept of the reflective practitioner (Scanlan & Chernomas 1997; Reason, 1994). Schön (1983) theorised that reflection facilitated the identification of one's 'theories in use' and that as a result of this activity new knowledge (previously embedded in practice) and theory could be generated. As such, other than offering examples of reflective activity, the primary aim of exemplars, narratives and so on, is an attempt to resonate experientially with a broad cross-section of readers. However, this is problematic in that all that is available to readers is the text – discrete, stylised and highly edited. What is never explicit is the writer's internal frame of reference, or their personal (or professional) values, beliefs and philosophies. We are not always privy to what motivates them and as such can never come to understand the environment that the encounter takes place in and, more crucially, can never fully understand the patients' perspective in all of this. In addition, few judgements of the gap between the practitioners espoused theories and their theories in use, can be made.

This is compounded by the fact that in presenting and reading articles in books or journals there is little, if any, opportunity for dialogue. The only reasonable use, then, for such narratives is as an example of how to write a reflective narrative. However, I think that it is more likely that this point is missed (the intention is not usually made explicit by the author) and that the narratives are held up as containing some kind of a 'nursing truth'. Be that as it may, what is known is that each reader approaches the text from the perspective of their own knowledge, experience and from within the context of the consensual reality of their own practice area.

There are, of course, examples of authors writing in reflective fashion about their own nursing practice. But always it seems they lack the confidence to allow their subjective experience to stand alone, peppered as these texts are with references to 'the literature' to ground, justify and validate. Constantly seeking to integrate their theory in use with established theories negates practitioners developing practice-based theory. This in turn prevents such texts from becoming truly emancipatory, and it seems reasonable to conclude that such writing is still shaped by the prevailing norms of scholarly discourse.

The ethical dilemma is inevitably complex and sensitive. Since Schön's (re)introduction of reflection there has been a proliferation of theories and models developed by, predominantly, nurse educationalists. For example, among the most commonly cited are Boud et al. (1985), Mezirow (1981) and Johns (1995). These writers are producing models and theories at a time when both nurse education and nursing practice have been influenced by a shift towards humanist philosophy (Playle, 1995; Hewison & Wildman, 1996; Hopton, 1997). Purdy (1997) asserts that humanist values and ideology have dominated education in particular. However, in the use of the narratives and vignettes mentioned above, there is a departure from the humanist foundations of Schön and an engagement in a facile reduction of the patient. This is perhaps best illustrated in this quote from bell hooks:

> Often this speech about the 'Other' annihilates, erases: 'no need to hear your voice when I can talk about you better than you can speak about yourself. No need to hear your voice. Only tell me about your pain. I want to know your story. And then I will tell it back to you in a new way. Tell it back to you in such a way that it has become mine, my own. Re-writing you, I write myself anew. I am still author, authority. I am still the colonizer, the speak subject, and you are now at the center of my talk. (1990: 151–2)

Unavoidably, and consistent with counselling technologies, it seems that we reduce the patient to the status of object, hardly humanist. Is there a solution? To regain the humanist ground inadvertently lost to such activity one would have to consider a more sophisticated discourse than a single viewpoint narrative. By this I mean that running parallel to the narrative of the author/practitioner would have to be a narrative by the patient/subject. This may promote balance and illuminate the patients' perspective, including not only the meaning of the singular encounter but also the meaning of the illness experience in their life. Is this solution realisable? Probably not. Is there an alternative?

An introduction to autoethnography

Autoethnography stands at the intersection of three genres of writing that are becoming increasingly visible, these being native anthropology, ethnic autobiography and autobiographical ethnography. The word 'autoethnography' has been used for at least two decades by literary critics as well as by anthropologists and sociologists and can have multiple meanings (Reed-Danahay, 1997). Like many other terms used by social scientists, the meanings and applications of autoethnography have evolved in a manner that makes precise definition and application difficult. The scope and variety of practices that come under the broad rubric of autoethnography is vast (see Ellis & Bochner, 2000, for a comprehensive account).

Essentially, autoethnography blurs distinctions between social science and literature, the personal and the social, the individual and culture, self and other, and researcher and subject (Ellis, 1998). It therefore offers nurses the opportunity to write about their experiences without the obligation to refer to theory for validation, for as a form of self-narrative that places the self within a social context it is both a method and a text (Reed-Danahay, 1997). The author's privilege personal stories over abstract theory and analysis allow and encourage alternative readings and multiple interpretations. They ask their readers to feel the truth of their stories and to become co-participants engaging in the storyline morally, emotionally, aesthetically and intellectually (Richardson, 1994).

Storytelling is fundamental to human experience. Through narration we make meaning out of experience and live within the stories we create. Personal stories can clash with cultural narratives that advocate appropriate or correct behaviour, that in turn provide versions of the way the world should be (Jago, 1996). As Bochner (1997a) points out, there is nothing as theoretical as a good story.

Autoethnography is most certainly not an easy option. There are powerful unwritten codes and conventions which individuals and the wider profession would have to relax with; in particular, the artificial boundary between person and professional (Freshwater, 1998). Again I return to Sally Gadow's (1993) belief that the view that there is a separate 'nurse self' aligns with the traditional values that tend to view nurse as professional. Within this the nurse is discouraged from becoming 'involved', overt emotions and feelings are discouraged. This persists despite the fact that the movement of humanist health has attempted to soften the distinction between the personal and the professional; professionals are encouraged to behave and think like persons. In this respect, autoethnography involves the study of ones own experience as a site for understanding the broader cultural context (Jago, 1996).

Autoethnography is grounded in personal life. Usually written in first person voice, it pays attention to physical feelings, thoughts and emotions and is profoundly introspective (Ellis & Bochner, 2000). It is dependent on being able to write well and the self-questioning it demands is extremely difficult. Honest autoethnography generates a lot of fears, doubts and emotional pain. There is, of course, vulnerability in revealing yourself, particularly in not being able to take back what you have written or in having any control in how readers interpret your work (Ellis & Bochner, 2000). However, you do come to understand yourself in deeper ways and with understanding of self comes understanding of others.

Autoethnography appears in a variety of forms. For example, short stories, poetry, fiction, novels, photographic essays, personal essays, journals, fragmented layered writing and social science prose. These texts feature concrete action, dialogue, emotion, embodiment, spirituality and self-consciousness, appearing as relational and institutional stories affected by history, social structure and culture. These in turn are dialectically revealed through action, feeling, thought and language (Ellis and Bochner, 2000).

What follows is an example of autoethnography; from what has been written thus far you will appreciate that it would not be in the spirit of autoethnography to preview or explain the writing in any depth. I will, however, briefly set the scene.

In common with Art Bochner (1997b), the death of my father caused a collision of two worlds within myself: the professional and the personal. I was forced to confront the large gulf that divides them. There is an enormous difference between a personal and a 'detached' professional experience. I was stunned to learn how tame the professional world is in comparison to my own lived experience. Much autoethnographic work falls under the broad rubric of loss narratives. It is hardly surprising, as an experience of loss shatters the meaningful world people have assembled for themselves (Ellis, 1998). For me, death represented a great big nothing, I had nothing to get a grip on, and death is the contrary of contraries. You see, you can have hot/cold, sound/silence, light/dark and so on. But life/death is very different. We may understand life, but what is death? As I mentioned, what follows is an excerpt from a much larger piece of writing that was an attempt by myself to make sense of my experience, to understand, manage and recover by creating an account that makes sense of loss. It is called 'Singing Into The Void' and formed part of a thesis submitted for a Masters Degree.

Singing Into The Void
Dying

How well I remember the phone call, Mums struggle to find the right words only to reach the bit where there is only one way of saying it: 'Eh, son ... it's your Dad, he's got cancer'. I don't remember much else, I was in a kind of daze, background noise just faded away and I stared out of the window at nothing. But I wasn't scared or afraid. Somehow I knew this was going to happen. I knew he'd been having the tests and I knew he had cancer. There was a certain inevitability about all of this.

Jenni can't understand why I'm not going to the textbooks. I'm a mental health nurse, I keep saying. She doesn't understand. She doesn't understand that all I need to know is that he's dying. I don't need to know about the disease in all its glory and I especially don't need to know about the treatment. I know where this thing goes, I know the end and that's all I need to know. Just so long as his pain control is good then I'll be OK. What I do need is to be there, to be a son to my parents and a brother to my brothers; I especially need to be available for Dad. Curiously all our family positions are suddenly clear and well defined again. I'm back to being Wee Roddy, the baby of the family.

I looked Allan right in the eye and said, 'Allan, he won't die in winter, he will die in springtime.' I believed this to be true, I have no idea why but as soon as Mum told me I just knew, I knew he would die in springtime. Allan said, 'Thanks bro, I needed to hear that, thanks.' He asked no questions, he just believed.

My trips down home are getting more frequent. Mum is struggling, and Allan. Jim seems OK, trying like crazy to keep everything normal, maybe to protect us all – hell, I don't know. What I do know is that this can't go on much longer. Everyone is telling him that he is going to make it, that he is going to get better. He is colluding, agreeing with them, trying to protect them. He knows fine well that he is dying and now he's getting worried because he thinks that he is the only one who is ready for it. It's just me and Mum and Dad in the house, Dad is lying through in bed. 'Mum, this can't go on, he needs to know that he is dying and he needs to know that we know.' I can't bear to tell him, she says. 'Then I'll do it.' She sighs, sad and relieved. In one of his wakeful moments I go to him. 'Dad, you know that you're not going to get better, don't you?' Silence. 'Don't you, Dad?' He looked me right in the eye and said, 'Thank God for that son, thank God for that.' I can hear Mum crying in the kitchen. 'Thank God for that,' he said again, 'Thanks son'. I ask if there is anything that he wants to talk about, anyone he needs to see, anything he needs to ask. He says that he needs to be on his own for a wee bit. He doesn't want to break down in front of me. He is relieved though, a tension, a weight, has left him. From this night on we can be together in openness, no secrets. Soon after that night he is admitted to the hospice. It's funny how we keep children away from the dying. I told Mum that I was taking Aidan and Niamh to visit Dad and she was horrified, but I'm nothing if not stubborn. He loved it; they were completely at peace with him. Niamh sitting on the bed beside him, Aidan playing snap with his big cousin Laura, they brightened up that day and that space. It was the last time he saw them and they him. I wrote this poem.

The Gene Pool

Your wasting thin arms
Can no longer support those big hands,
Big hands, firm grip.
So they lie, tapping a gentle rhythm
On the bed sheets.

White sheets folded
And tucked tight across your chest,
Afraid you might fly away?
But you'll stay a while yet.
A faint smile lightens your grey pained face, as,

Lying in your nest of pillows
You watch in delight
As the gene pool, plays
At the foot of your bed.

While Dad was dying I had my moments. But only once have I cried like I was going to dissolve. When he went to the hospice we thought that he wouldn't see Christmas – so much for springtime. But he rallied; we underestimated the effect of good care and his desire to be at home with Betty. And then the sudden rapid slip backwards. For some reason they don't think that he needs palliative care now and he is admitted to a remote geriatric hospital. In the middle of nowhere, nowhere near home, a run-down dilapidated, low morale, no future, no hope kind of a place. I went to see him there, chanted my mantra that the staff try hard in difficult circumstances. It hurt like hell as I tried to switch off my nurse head going in there. I went to visit him alone in that place. He was lying to attention, head barely on the pillows, more alone than I had ever seen him. The sights, sounds and smells around him would have at one time horrified him. He lay there staring at the discoloured, cracked painted ceiling, mouth open, a melted ice cream just out of reach: and I loved him more profoundly in that moment than I have ever loved anything.

'Ah, hullo,' he said, in his new-found quiet, tender voice, the steady grip of his big handshake straight from his big heart. 'So how are you,' I asked, an attempt at normality, a no-risk question. 'Well, I can't complain, I've had a good life and a wonderful family.' I crumbled, he turned to look at the ceiling, not wanting to embarrass me I suspect. He sleeps, he wakes. I have composed myself; he asks for the family, for Jenni and the wee ones. He sleeps, he wakes. 'Ah, hullo, when did you come,' the firm grip. We talk some more and then he sleeps again, deeper. I kiss his forehead and leave, a now well-established ritual. I had planned to speak to a nurse but during the hour or so I spent with him I had seen none. No angels swooping about in white – why the catheter, was it in-dwelling (I didn't look, he wouldn't have liked that), why the major tranquillisers, did they know he'd been like that six months ago and it was because he had hypercalcemia, how was his pain control, his eating … But I didn't ask. I didn't ask because I couldn't speak. I sat in the car in the hospital car park and cried for about an hour.

Relief. Dad's back in the hospice, thanks to Mum and the Minister. The Minister had asked why Dad wasn't transferred back to the hospice, the staff said 'because the family haven't asked' – so much for primary nursing! Mum wanted me to do the asking. I said no because for some reason I felt it was important for her to deal with this. Mum did it and did it well. He was transferred back there five days before he died. Five days of rest, of comfort, of peace, of dignity, of pain relief – of care. Only one more time did I get the 'Ah, hullo,' the firm grip from the heart and a last talk. I asked what hymns did he want, he just looked away. 'My Dad would have been disappointed in me that I stopped going to church,' he said. We talk. I reassure him that he had been a good man, a good husband and a good father. I reassured him that the most important thing of all was that church or not, he had lived his values, Christian values. I was honest, I told him that sure there were moments when I had despised him, his rules and his values, but now a bit older and a bit wiser and with children of my own I appreciated more than ever those lessons, hard as they were at the time. Finally, I told him that these were the values and the parenting I hoped to pass on to the kids. He thanked me for speaking honestly to him. We picked three hymns.

The Death

Ann-Marie is on duty – we used to dance together. She asked to talk. 'I'm going to give him a suppository, Roddy, you know what that means?' 'Yeh, sure I do,' I said. 'Do you want to tell your family or will I?' she asked. 'No, I'll do it.' I tell them, they understand fine, Mum, Allan, Jim, Joan, Aunt Anne and Uncle John. Ann-Marie comes in, 'Roddy do you want to help?' 'I'd love to, Ann-Marie.' My last memory of Dad alive is of me cradling him in my arms while Ann-Marie gives him the suppository. Looking into his eyes speaking loud to reassure him because I don't think he saw me, but he understood the word 'Dad'. I held a life in that moment; cradled in my arms. I was happy in that moment. At 1.50 a.m. on Tuesday the 21st of April 1998, my Dad breathed out and didn't breathe back in. Springtime.

Ah, Jim, Jim ... Never have I heard so much love being invested in a three-letter word. She said it in a rhythm, a chant, and stroked his cheek gently as if he might object – as he used to, for he was not one for public displays of affection. But he didn't flinch. He allowed it to happen. Over 50 years of love, and regrets; spoken in a three-letter word, Jim.

The last time I saw him he was lying in his coffin – no more firm grip. But the kissing the forehead ritual continued. I can still feel the chill on my lips.

Implications for practice

Our attitude toward death and dying, perhaps more than any other single phenomena we are likely to encounter, shape our own individual experience. Developing an understanding of our own attitudes and beliefs will go a long way to assisting us in being present for those who are dying and for those who have been bereaved. It is therefore essential that we learn to value our life experiences, and while I have used the example of death, dying and bereavement, I do of course extend this principle to all of our life experiences and therefore to any counselling situation.

Here the medical model with its objective/descriptive stance and its model of assessment and diagnosis of grief and bereavement in stages is not useful. It is not useful because it pathologises grief. One of the problems with grieving being conceptualised as a model is that just as our losses are unique to each of us, so are our ways of responding and coping with loss. This is a crucial point given that the majority of counselling models are intended to facilitate an individuals' passage through these 'stages'. People do not universally respond to the same emotional 'cues' in the same way, nor is the experience of feeling an emotion the same for all groups. This is true even within a group or society (Tarlow, 1999; Cox, 2000) and as a principle is a good example of the failings of cognitivism's computational metaphor.

My experience led me to understand that the world seen in terms of intellectual concepts might appear simple and easy to put to rights, but the complexity of the reality is always too great. In bereavement there are no stages, there is no blueprint and grief is not sequential. Stopping the feelings does not ease the person's pain; we have to adjust our capacity to tolerate another person's pain and in this the nurse needs to learn to live in a startlingly familiar 'conceptual' space that demands emotional openness. That space turns out to be the space of everyday practical life.

It is in this space that the nurse needs to be able to draw upon all of their life experience, to truly and fully understand their values and their beliefs and to access these as a whole person and as a source of strength that will allow them to be fully present for the other, the person in need. The medical model has, perhaps inadvertently, disallowed the passion of grief and the fact that people are on a journey: someone has to be prepared to go on that journey with them.

In conclusion

As practitioners we have at our disposal a variety of tools to help us construct meaning including painting, drawing, photography, reflective reading and writing be it biography, poetry, journals or stories. These tools, and in particular narrative, are a means to progress philosophically congruent practice, either as an approach or in conjunction with counselling which honours the personal and includes ordinariness and self-awareness within the application of therapeutic use of self. Counselling in the absence of these qualities and values is a technology and incongruous with holism.

Toni Vezeau (1994) defines narrative as being a representation of a personal reality, and so in sharing my narratives I engage in a confessional act. As Rose writes:

In confessing one is objectified by another ... but in confessing one constitutes oneself. In the act of speaking, through the obligation to produce words that are true to an inner reality, through the self-examination that precedes and accompanies speech, one becomes a subject for oneself. (1994: 244)

In sharing my story I continue to construct the story of my life and in doing so construct myself. In so doing, however, I hope that something I share will resonate with you and that we make some kind of connection. Telling any narrative in any setting is a bridging performance, it connects the teller and the listener and in so doing, their lives. When stories are withheld we are deprived from gaining direct and intimate knowledge of collective experiences. When stories are shared it creates a sense of belonging and community. This sense of belonging and of community is a powerful way of enabling us to transform self and practice, to change the story for self and others, and has massive healing potential.

References

Apple M. (1988) *Teachers and Texts: A Political Economy of Class and Gender Relations in Education*. New York: Routledge.
Barton, A.J. (2000) 'Reflection: nursing's practice and education panacea?' *Journal of Advanced Nursing*, **31** (5), 1009–1017.
Bochner, A.P. (1997a) 'Storied lives: recovering the moral importance of social theory' in J.S. Trent (ed.) *At the Helm in Speech Communication*. Boston: Allyn and Bacon.
Bochner, A.P. (1997b) 'It's About Time: Narrative and the Divided Self'. *Qualitative Inquiry*, **3** (4), 418–38.
Boud, D., Keogh, K. & Walker, D. (1985) *Reflection: Turning Experience into Learning*. London: Kogan Page.

Carr, E.C.J. (1996) 'Reflecting on clinical practice: hectoring talk or reality?' *Journal of Clinical Nursing,* **5,** 289–95.

Cody, W.K. (2000) 'Paradigm Shift or Paradigm Drift? A Meditation on Commitment and Transcendence'. *Nursing Science Quarterly,* **13** (2), 93–102.

Cowling, W.R. (2000) 'Healing as Appreciating Wholeness'. *Advanced nursing science,* **22** (3), 16–32.

Cox, G.R. (2000) 'Children, Spirituality and Loss'. *Illness, Crisis and Loss,* **8** (1), 60–70.

Ellis C. (1998) 'Exploring Loss through Auto ethnographic inquiry: Auto ethnographic Stories, Co-Constructed Narratives, and Interactive Interviews' in Harvey, J.H. (ed.) *Perspectives on Loss: A Sourcebook.* London: Brunner Mazel.

Ellis, C. & Bochner, A.P. (2000) 'Auto ethnography, Personal Narrative, Reflexivity'. In Denzin, N. & Lincoln, Y. *Handbook of Qualitative Research,* 2nd edn. London: Sage.

Fee, D. (2000) *Pathology And The Postmodern: Mental illness as discourse and experience.* London: Sage.

Freshwater, D. (1998) 'Transformatory Learning in Nurse Education'. Unpublished PhD Thesis. University of Nottingham.

Freshwater, D. & Johns, C. (2001) 'Global Communities of Caring and Beyond: An integrative model for nursing practice?' Keynote paper presented at 23rd Research Conference of the International Association for Human Caring. Stirling University.

Freshwater, D. & Rolfe, G. (2001) 'Critical Reflexivity: A politically and ethically engaged research method for nursing'. *NTResearch,* **6** (1), 526–37.

Gadow, S. (1993) 'Existential Advocacy' cited in Watson, J. (1993) *A Theory of Human Caring in Nursing: Topical Bibliography.* Book for Course Participants. Center for Human Caring, University of Colorado School of Nursing and Scottish Highlands Centre for Human Caring, Highland & Western Isles College of Nursing.

Haggman-Laitila, A. (1997) 'Health as an individuals way of existence'. *Journal of Advanced Nursing,* **25**: 1, 45–53.

Hewison, A. & Wildman, S. (1996) 'The theory–practice gap in nursing: a new dimension'. *Journal of Advanced Nursing,* **24**: 4,754–61.

Hiraki, A. (1992) 'Tradition, rationality and power in Introductory Nursing Text Books: A Critical Hermeneutics Study'. *Advanced Nursing Science,* **14** (3), 1–12.

Heath, H. & Freshwater, D. (2000) 'Clinical Supervision as Emancipatory Process: Avoiding inappropriate intent'. *Journal of Advanced Nursing,* **32** (3), 1298–1306.

hooks, b. (1990) 'Talking back: Thinking feminist, thinking black'. Boston: South End, in Denzin, N.K. & Lincoln, Y.S. (1994) (eds) *Handbook of Qualitative Research.* London: Sage.

Hopps, L.C. (1994) 'The development of research in the United Kingdom'. *Journal of Clinical Nursing,* **3**: 4, 199–204.

Hopton, J. (1997) 'Towards a critical theory of mental health nursing'. *Journal of Advanced Nursing,* **25**: 3, 492–500.

Horsefall, J.M. (1995) 'Madness in our methods: nursing research and scientific epistemology'. *Nursing Inquiry,* **2** (1), 2–9.

Jago, B.J. (1996) 'Postcards, Ghosts and Fathers: Revising Family Stories'. *Qualitative Inquiry,* **2** (4), 495–516.

Jaspers, K. (1948) in Sartre, J.P. (1948) *Existentialism and Humanism* (Philip Mairet, trans.) London: Methuen.

Johns, C. (1995) 'Framing learning through reflection within Carper's fundamental ways of knowing in nursing'. *Journal of Advanced Nursing,* **22**: 2, 226–34.

Johnson, M.B. (1990) 'The holistic paradigm in nursing: the diffusion of an innovation'. *Research Nursing Health*, **13**, 129–39. Cited in Newman, M.A. (1992) 'Prevailing Paradigms in Nursing'. *Nursing Outlook*, **40** (1), 10–13.

Kolcaba, R. (1997) 'The primary holisms in nursing'. *Journal of Advanced Nursing*, **25**: 2, 290–96.

Kuhn, T. (1970) *The structure of scientific revolutions*. Chicago: University of Chicago Press.

Mezirow, J. (1981) 'A critical theory of adult learning and adult education'. *Adult Education*, **32** (1), 3–24.

Mitchell, G.J. & Cody, W.K. (1993) 'The Role of Theory in Qualitative Research'. *Nursing Science Quarterly*, **6** (4), 170–78.

Okri, B. (1997) *A Way of Being Free*. London: Pheonix House.

Oldnall, A. (1996) 'A critical analysis of nursing: meeting the spiritual needs of patients'. *Journal of Advanced Nursing*, **23**: 1, 138–44.

Parse, R.R. (2001) 'Language and the Sow-Reap Rhythm'. *Nursing Science Quarterly*, **14** (4), 273.

Picard, C. (2000) 'Who are you and what are you doing? Embodied nursing praxis to transform practice and research' in Freshwater, D. (2000) (ed.) *Making a Difference*. Portsmouth: Nursing Praxis International.

Pickering, J. (1997) *The Authority of Experience*. Richmond: Curzon.

Playle, J.F. (1995) 'Humanism and positivism in nursing: contradictions and conflicts'. *Journal of Advanced Nursing*, **22**: 1, 979–84.

Powers, B.A. & Knapp, T.R. (1990) *A Dictionary of Nursing Theory and Research*. London: Sage.

Pullen, L., Tuck, I. & Mix, K. (1996) 'Mental Health Nurses Spiritual Perspectives'. *Journal of Holistic Nursing,* **14** (2), 85–97.

Purdy, M. (1997) 'Humanist ideology and nurse education. 2. Limitations of humanist educational theory in nurse education'. *Nurse Education Today*, **17**: 3, 196–202.

Reason, P. (1994) 'Three Approaches to Participative Inquiry' in Denzin, N.K. & Lincoln, Y.S. (eds) (1994) *Handbook of Qualitative Research*. London: Sage, p. 324–39.

Reed-Danahay, D.E. (1997) *Auto/Ethnography: Rewriting the Self and the Social*. Oxford: Berg.

Richardson, L. (1994). 'Writing: A Method of Inquiry' in Denzin, N.K. & Lincoln, Y.S. (1994) (eds) *Handbook of Qualitative Research*. London: Sage.

Rolfe, G. (1998) *Expanding Nursing Knowledge*. Oxford: Butterworth Heinemann.

Rolfe, G. (1996) *Closing the Theory-Practice Gap. A new paradigm for nursing*. Oxford: Butterworth Heinemann.

Rolfe, G., Freshwater, D. & Jasper, M. (2001) *Critical Reflection for Nursing and the Helping Professions*. Basingstoke: Palgrave.

Rose, N. (1994) *Governing the Soul* London: Routledge. Cited in Crowe, M. (1998) 'The power of the word: some post-structural considerations of qualitative approaches in nursing research'. *Journal of Advanced Nursing*, **28** (2), 339–44.

Sarter, B. (1988) 'Philosophic sources of nursing theory'. *Nursing Science Quarterly*, **1** (2), 52–9. Cited in Newman, M.A. (1992) 'Prevailing Paradigms in Nursing'. *Nursing Outlook*, **40** (1), 10–13.

Scanlan, J.M. & Chernomas, W.M. (1997) 'Developing the reflective teacher'. *Journal of Advanced Nursing,* **25**: 6, 1138–43.

Schön, D.A. (1983) *The Reflective Practitioner*. Aldershot: Avebury.

Schön, D.A. (1987) *Educating the Reflective Practitioner*. London: Jossey Bass.

Seedhouse, D. (2000) *Practical Nursing Philosophy: The Universal Ethical Code*. Chichester: John Wiley.

Tarlow, S. (1999) *Bereavement and Commemoration: An Archaeology of Mortality*. Oxford: Blackwell Science.

Taylor, B. (1992) 'From helper to human: a reconceptualization of the nurse as person'. *Journal of Advanced Nursing*, **17**: 9, 1042–9.

Teilhards, de Chardin, P. (1959) *The Phenomenon of Man*. Collins, London. Cited in O'Donohue, N. (1993) *The Mountain Behind The Mountain. Aspects of the Celtic Tradition*. Edinburgh: T. and T. Clark.

Vaughan, B. (1987) 'Bridging the gap'. *Senior Nurse*, **6** (5), 30–31.

Vezeau, T. (1994) 'Narrative inquiry in nursing' in Chinn, P. & Watson, J. (eds.) *Art and Aesthetics in Nursing*. New York: National League for Nursing Press.

Watson, J. (1999) *Postmodern Nursing and Beyond*. London: Churchill Livingstone.

3 Therapeutic Nursing and Technology: Clinical Supervision and Reflective Practice in a Critical Care Setting

Jill Down

The advent of reflective practice and the recommendations for clinical supervision (NHS ME, 1993; UKCC, 1996) provide an opportunity for exploring and developing practice using practical experiences whilst encouraging personal growth to improve patient care (Butterworth & Faugier, 1994). The argument for learning through experience is supported by the writings of Patricia Benner (1984; Benner et al., 1992; Benner et al., 1999) and work with critical care nurses that supports the view that practitioners base actions on previous experiences rather than text-book knowledge.

There have been an increasing number of technological and scientific advances within critical care during the last two decades. These advances have been reflected in the changing role of the critical care nurse with an emphasis on managing complex mechanical and pharmacological interventions. Coupled with the management of extended workloads and staff shortages within already restricted finances, it is not surprising that the focus of nursing and caring gets lost within the biomedical emphasis. The advent of clinical supervision centred on reflective practice has promoted a refocusing of the emphasis towards patient-centred care and caring as central to nursing as described by Watson (1988a). It provides a structure within which any nurse can develop both personally and professionally, maximising their therapeutic potential to improve patient care whilst balancing the technology with caring.

This chapter focuses on a personal experience of clinical supervision using guided reflective practice to illustrate the process and the integration of research-based theories together with theories based on experience. It illustrates the importance of clinical supervision to challenge practice within a supportive environment enabling enlightenment, empowerment and emancipation of the practitioner and their therapeutic potential (Fay, 1987). It also highlights the active commitment that is required for both therapeutic nursing and to the furtherance of practical nursing knowledge.

The examples used in this chapter are drawn from my own experience of receiving clinical supervision that had a profound effect on my personal and professional life, providing a window through which to view my practice, highlighting the need to know myself in order to be of therapeutic use to the patient and their families. The impact of the experience has transformed my practice and celebrates nursing as therapy, as something to be cherished and nurtured, specifically within the critical care setting.

Contextual considerations

Much of the work has been derived from a research project in which I utilised a formal structure, that of philosophical framing within a phenomenological method (Johns, 1998). In describing some of the tensions nurses encounter in their everyday practice, which reflect the 'swampy lowlands' that Schön (1987) portrays, I reflect upon the dilemmas, the thought processes and interactions of the lived experience of caring for a critically ill patient, attempting to seek out the deeper meaning of the therapeutic encounter. Munhall (1994) asserts that as nurses we should be looking for methods of research which can find a place in mainstream literature, written in conversational, informal style that are rigidly bound by methods. Narrative is used to enlarge the vision of particular experiences and allows a weaving of human context and responses which provide a solid base for the development of nursing knowledge (Younger, 1990). It seeks to explore a phenomenon with the discovery of salient questions with reflection and openness to a situation, rather than discovering measurable parts–it is not the intent of narrative to produce theory (Vezeau, 1994). Stories have long been used to convey nurses' knowledge of individuals to each other and have always been part of how we explore the shared world of our patients. It has helped develop our personal knowledge rooted in clinical practice (Boykin & Schoenhofer, 1991). Vezeau (1994) suggests that storytellers undergo personal epistemological processes as they pursue a story and an authentic story will demonstrate the depth and breadth of human conditions within specific contexts, whilst also developing aesthetic knowing of individual situations. Benner (1991) describes two forms of narrative and says that liberation narratives depict nurses 'finding their voice'. This is valuable in enabling nurses to discover their own care giving and indeed therapeutic worth in a world dominated by high technology. Mischler (1986) notes that telling stories is a significant way for individuals to give meaning to and express their understanding of their experience. Stories, then, have a therapeutic value of their own, both for the orator and for the listener (Frank, 2000).

   The reflection presented in this chapter focuses on my experience of caring for Jennie and personal and professional issues surrounding her care. I concentrate on the issues that were raised within supervision and which both my supervisor and myself considered of most significance. The physiology of the illness and definition of the treatments are described only to enable comprehension of the situation and are not intended to provide in-depth clinical knowledge. The story is presented as a *whole* story and as it was written in my reflective diary. Subsequent analysis allows further exploration of clinical considerations, the implications for nursing practice arising from these and an integration of theoretical principles related to nursing, caring and therapy.

Description of the experience

Jennie, a 22-year-old student, was admitted to intensive care in extremis with meningococcal septicaemia. She had felt 'under the weather' for only two days whilst visiting her parents before collapsing and requiring maximal support for multi-organ failure. She required full respiratory support via a ventilator, circulatory support with catecholamines and renal support using haemodiafiltration. She was so unstable for the first five days that it was a constant challenge and we were uncertain from one minute to the next as to whether she would survive. She had no circulation to her legs from mid-calf, no circulation to her hands from her forearms and her digits were black. She had required fasciotomies to relieve the pressure within her calf and forearm muscles. At this time, Jennie's appearance was very unpleasant. She was covered in blue/black areas that rendered her unrecognisable to her family. My first meeting with Jennie was six days after her admission; I was to look after her for the duration of my shift and received handover from Jennie's nurse at the bedside.

Personal feelings in this situation

I have seen many harrowing sights during my career in ICU but I was horrified by the sight of this young girl covered in necrotic black areas all over her body. Her extremities were now 'mummified' and I struggled to see the person beyond the 'blackness' and the banks of machinery. I felt overwhelming sadness as I was told of the extent of the damage to Jennie's limbs, which were discreetly covered. My sadness encompassed feelings for Jennie, her family and the whole situation. In addition I felt guilt that I was part of a system which was able to prolong life with such seemingly horrible consequences. At that moment I regretted working in an ICU setting; I was surprised by the intensity of the feelings I was experiencing. Handover was an emotive event, the nurse giving me information was obviously saddened and near to tears when describing the extent of the damage to limbs and the multi-organ support Jennie was requiring. There was much shaking of heads by staff. The feeling of the nurses on the ICU was, without exception, that 'we wished she had died or would die'. It was too unbearable to consider this previously fit, healthy and attractive young woman looking like this and contemplating her future. We were overwhelmed by the awfulness of the situation and on more than one occasion nurses stated that they would not want to live if it were they in the bed. There was relief expressed by a few nurses that they did not need to look after Jennie since it meant they did not need to confront their own beliefs and could, to some extent, distance themselves from the emotional labour (Freshwater, 1998; Menzies, 1988).

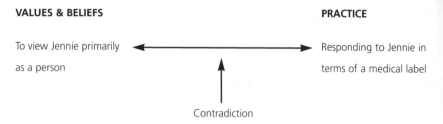

Figure 3.1   *Contradiction in attitude towards Jennie; model based on Johns (1998)*

The shift was a busy one; I seemed to be caring for the technology rather than a human being. The amount of drug and mechanical support required to maintain Jennie meant that I was endlessly making up infusions, titrating inotropes, balancing fluids with haemodiafiltration and performing dressings normally done in the theatre situation. I also needed to acknowledge the presence of Jennie's family, which required a substantial amount of my energy, whilst I was simultaneously caring for Jennie. I felt physically and emotionally drained when handing over to the nurse on the night duty.

I had been unable to touch her because of her poor skin condition and the plethora of interventions and was desperate to find someway to connect to what felt like an object in the bed. I was also trying to connect with my therapeutic capacity. I decided I would ask Jennie's family if Jennie used 'scrunchies' in her hair – her hair was long and blond – as using one would help me solve the dilemma of being unable to touch her and help regain some sense of her humanness.

As I reflected on the situation I began to question myself and why I felt so strongly that Jennie's life would not be worth living without part of or all of her limbs. How could I begin to put myself in her position? Was it right that I should try? All my answers were borne out of irrational emotional responses and I sensed that I needed to resolve these issues in order to nurse Jennie humanistically. This preliminary reflection highlighted the incongruence of my values and beliefs and my practice, so I mentally highlighted the contradiction (see Figure 3.1).

The next shift

I went back to work the next morning to look after Jennie and started to feel differently about her. I felt more positive despite being surrounded by the still 'shaking heads' and negative feelings of other nurses. It was now seven days since her admission and it was necessary to make uncomfortable decisions regarding further treatment for Jennie. She still required respiratory support, renal support, was septic and had questionable neurological status – she was unconscious, despite no sedation, and had nonviable lower legs and hands. She was not improving at all. I took all her dressings down for the consultant plastic surgeon to review them before he, the ICU consultant and three junior doctors began to discuss Jennie and her future. I was not invited to join them. I felt very strongly that I wanted to be part of the decision-making process and asked the nurse in charge to relieve me so that I could join the doctors. I did not give her the opportunity to refuse!

The discussion was in progress when I entered the room, but I was not acknowledged and the flow of the conversation continued. The group of professionals were discussing the likelihood of Jennie's recovery; the plastic consultant was explaining the nature of the drastic surgery required to remove all the necrotic tissue. He had never before encountered such extensive problems during his career and he was giving us his opinion based on the surgical techniques available. I took the opportunity to ask him several technical questions about the state of the limbs to satisfy myself that I was informed – I had intimate knowledge of how they looked but not the technical knowledge to understand the implications. At this point he moved so that I was physically within the group. He acknowledged that I had knowledge about the wounds and their care and was able to give him information about the state of areas on the underside of her body. Jennie would require removal of her legs, initially through the knees, and of one hand and digits from another, with much additional surgery beyond this.

The discussion continued, led mainly by the ICU consultant; it was evident that Jennie was not getting better despite our best efforts. She remained in multi-organ failure and a search of the available literature revealed no record of anyone surviving this disease with such injuries as she had. The discussion centred on the withdrawal of treatment, as it appeared from our debate that Jennie had been offered all the treatments available with no obvious improvement. The only remaining treatment option, which might possibly help, was to remove Jennie's necrotic limbs. Whilst taking part in these discussions I was suddenly struck by the feeling that we should not be discussing withdrawal of treatment and needed to vocalise my concerns:

> I'm not sure that I feel comfortable discussing withdrawal of treatment. I feel it is being discussed because the alternative requires us to mutilate Jennie's body extensively. If we were talking about Jennie who was tetraplegic as a result of injuries, I don't think we would be taking the same stance.

My comments were followed by a silence. In that moment I felt very sure that we should not withdraw treatment and had transcended my emotional feelings to acknowledge my real values. If removing the limbs gave Jennie a chance a life, it was not for us to speculate or impose our feelings onto her. I was unsure of the response I would receive from the doctors, but felt able to assert my views. In the event, the ICU consultant looked at me and thanked me for my comment. He said that it had helped to put things into context and that I had used a very valid point, which we had previously been in danger of missing. I was surprised to be thanked. I did not believe that the doctors truly considered that withdrawal of treatment was a real option but felt the need to vocalise my thoughts. It was agreed that we should proceed with the surgery to give Jennie a chance, whilst acknowledging that she may still not survive and that there was a long struggle ahead of us all. I came out of the room to look after Jennie again

PHILOSOPHICAL FRAMING	Confronting and clarifying the beliefs/values that constitute desirable practice.
ROLE FRAMING	Clarifying role boundaries/relationships/ legitimate authority and power to act within practice.
THEORETICAL FRAMING	Assimilating theory and research findings with personal knowing.
REALITY PERSPECTIVE FRAMING	Acknowledging that practising in new ways is not necessarily easy – whilst helping the practitioner to become knowledgeable and empowered to take necessary action.
PROBLEM FRAMING	Focuses problem identification and resolution that emerge within experience.
TEMPORAL FRAMING	This recognises how reflection is not an isolated event but connected through experiences over time and anticipating future experiences.
FRAMING THE DEVELOPMENT OF EFFECTIVENESS	Clearly it is essential that adequate ways of monitoring growth of effectiveness are constructed and implemented; ideally this should be done by the practitioner within the growth of their professional responsibility.

Figure 3.2   *Framing perspectives; based on Johns' model (1997)*

and explained to the other nurses what had been decided; this was difficult as I was faced with their disbelief at what was proposed but remained very sure it was the right decision.

Framing perspectives

> In trying to find meaning in our lives and to make sense of the things that happen to us, we seek frameworks of understanding that we can impose on the bewildering chaos of our existence. (Brookfield, 1987: 45)

There are many issues raised within this reflection and to make sense of them in the context of therapeutic nursing, a framing technique will be used (see Figure 3.2). This replicates the structure of challenging and supporting offered by supervision and focuses on the problem identification and resolution that emerge from the experience.

Implications for therapeutic practice

What follows is a detailed reflection on the experience of caring for Jennie using the framing perspectives model, highlighting the implications of this for therapeutic nursing practice.

Philosophical Framing

As previously stated, caring is central to nursing (Watson, 1988a; Watson, 1988b) and to my personal beliefs, caring for Jennie in this clinical situation caused me to challenge, confront and clarify what I understood by the concept of caring and caring in a technologically dominated environment.

I seemed unable to focus on Jennie as a fellow human; her appearance was alien and she was diminished by the presence of much technological equipment. However, I was aware of this and sought to confront the problem by suggesting combing Jennie's hair and using a 'scrunchie'. My feelings might be attributed to my training (in which the biomedical model was used) together with my long-term work in ICU, promoting a disposition to the technical rationality approach to knowledge (Schön, 1987). A more likely reason would be that this response was a coping mechanism on my part, protecting myself against involvement in what was a very difficult situation. This reflects the findings of May (1991), who showed that nurses feared the stresses that investing in a patient can bring and I had witnessed the feelings of relief by other nurses when they would not have to care for Jennie. May's (1991) findings are disputed by Morse (1991), who says that being involved and engaged with patients can be beneficial and help prevent burnout. Morse (1991) used ICU nurses as part of her study investigating nurse – patient relationships and identified four types of relationships. They ranged from clinical→therapeutic→connected→over-involved.

Whilst aspiring to being connected, that is viewing the patient primarily as a person and secondly as a patient, on reflection I became aware that I was initially using the professional, clinical relationship in order to depersonalise the patient (Morse, 1991). I remember trying not to look at a photograph of Jennie at her graduation whilst caring for her because it emphasised that she was a person beneath the awful exterior. Morse (1991) also suggests that if the nurse is committed to treatment goals or to the cure, these objectives may take priority over humanistic goals and she will be more likely to work within high-tech settings such as critical care. I acknowledged such traits in some colleagues and challenged myself to acknowledge the humanistic and therapeutic goals of nursing via reflection and supervision.

Cooper (1993), building on Rays (1987) seminal research on the phenomenon of care within ICU, proposes that it is a moral challenge for ICU nurses to confront the dehumanising impact of technology on nurse and patient. Without the caring relationship both nurse and patient are reduced to the status of objects – the nurse as an objective, competent technologist and the patient as an object to

| | FOCUS | |
Patient focused		Self focused
First Level Engaged		**Anti engaged**
Reflexive responses Connected response		Reflected response
EXPERIENCE		
Second Level **Pseudo engaged**		**Anti engaged**
Learned responses Professional response		Detached response

Figure 3.3   *Caregiver response by focus and experience; adapted from Morse et al. (1992: 810)*

be examined and evaluated. Ray described 'technological caring' as occurring within a moral realm, with the nurse blending technological competence with moral experiences and moral principles. Both Benner et al. (1992) and Ray (1987) have described how the union between technological competence and care can be enacted by expert nurses in ways that enrich human experience. Cooper's (1993) study highlights the need to bridge the paradox between cure and care and the objective values of science and the subjective values of human wellbeing. She suggests that nurses should be 'in tune' with technology, the patient and themselves, as they are the mediators between the technology which holds the potential for cure and the totality of the patient's needs. Further research describes nurses' responses to patients' suffering. Morse et al. (1992) suggest that the level of engagement with a patient is affected by whether the nurse is focused on herself or on the sufferer and whether the nurse is responding reflexively or with a learned response (see Figure 3.3).

Morse et al. (1992) note that observing a patient's suffering evokes an empathetic insight, which in turn evokes reflexive and spontaneous expressions – first level. However, they also acknowledge that constant exposure to patient suffering emotionally drains the practitioner and is therefore controlled by them to enable:

- the nurse to leave the distressed patient and move on and care for other patients; and
- the nurse to limit her involvement in the patient's suffering to avoid becoming emotionally drained and exhausted.

In clinical supervision using a reflective framework I was able to see that some nurses avoided Jennie by way of limiting their emotional involvement, establishing a first level anti-engagement response. At a personal level I believe I was struggling between the first level patient-focused response and at the second level I learned response of anti-engagement. It was extremely painful to use the reflexive response continually in the work with Jennie; it is emotionally draining and requires the expenditure of more energy than learned responses. Morse et al. (1992) contend that first level responses are always appropriate since they are evoked reflexively, but acknowledge that other responses are often appropriate since they protect the nurse.

The work of Ramos (1992) describes most accurately the level of my initial involvement with Jennie. It can be described as 'instrumental' and predominantly resembled sympathy and as such hampers the therapeutic relationship, what Ramos describes as 'paralysis'. It is interesting to note that this was the general experience on the ICU, with nurses feeling an overwhelming sense of pain and helplessness: 'we wished she was dead or would die' as it was too terrible to consider her life otherwise. Fortunately, I moved through levels one and two to level three; the shift in the level of involvement occurred during discussion with the doctors when I vocalised my feelings about of the nature of the discussions. It comprised of cognitive and emotional identification with the patient with some emotional identification and isolation of personal feelings. In supervision I described a feeling of 'transcending my emotional feelings and feeling extremely positive'; an understanding of my own personal responses helped to provide insight into the problems of always trying to practice according to personal beliefs in a critical care setting. Personal knowing is vital if one is to enable therapeutic use of self (Carper, 1978) and is necessary in order to be 'connected' with the situation. Where feelings may be negative towards others and block or hinder the nurse's therapeutic response, it can be seen as particularly useful to examine one's personal ways of knowing through reflection on action (Johns, 1993).

Marks-Maran and Rose's (1997) analogy of a cube to represent the many facets of nursing and nursing knowledge proved to be a valuable source of reflection in that it emphasises the complementarity of technological and human aspects of caring within an intensive care setting, rather than placing them in a hierarchical and oppositional relationship.

Role Framing

The doctor–nurse relationship
Clinical supervision encouraged me to embark upon an in-depth exploration of the doctor–nurse relationship within this clinical situation; I particularly reflected on my experience of not being invited to join the team in their discussions surrounding Jennie's treatment. Why did I have to ask the nurse in charge to relieve me to enable participation? In considering why the ICU consultant and his colleagues thought they could have full discussions and decision making about Jennie without a nursing input, I was provoked into examining the nurse–doctor relationship from a historical perspective with specific emphasis on the therapeutic role of the nurse in critical care.

Historically female nurses have taken on subordinate, non-professional roles within a male dominated medical division of labour (Wright, 1985) and it remains a struggle for them to assert their professional knowledge within this arena. Gamarnikov (in Sweet & Norman, 1995: 165) indicates that gender divisions are of pivotal importance in role assignment and of relationships between doctors and nurses drawing parallels with traditional family roles: the women (nurse) looking after the physical and emotional environment whilst the male (doctor) deciding what the really important work is and how it should be done. Going back to the Crimean War and to Florence Nightingale, Porter (1991) quotes her as saying that the nurse's role was to assist the doctor and provide a hygienic and comfortable environment. Perhaps at this point in history, bearing in mind the social context, the subordination of the nurse did not seem to pose particular problems; Keddy et al. (1986), for example, report the fact that in the 1920s and 1930s doctors were responsible for the recruitment and education of nurses, and good care was equated with following doctors orders. Maybe the nurses of that era were engaged in some sort of power game, just as they continue to be today?

The doctor–nurse game

Stein (1978) describes how nurses learn to give advice or show initiative whilst appearing to bow to the doctors' authority; he calls this the 'doctor–nurse game'. Stein suggests that open confrontation with authority figures is avoided, which obviously has a detrimental impact on the communication between professionals and consequently on patient care (Wright, 1985). The game, he argues, has arisen from the differences in the two trainings; he goes on to explain that doctors suffer anxiety because a mistake in treatment can have drastic consequences and as such doctors have difficulty in coming to terms with their fallibility. Instead they cultivate a sense of omnipotence that hampers their relationships with other professionals, particularly those with nurses. Porter (1991) suggests the nurses' position of having to cooperate in the facade of hiding their degree of skills, knowledge and information is a subservient position, which can be called 'informal covert decision making'. When Stein (1978) wrote his paper, nurse training was perhaps characterised by discipline and subservience, however, recent developments mean that practitioners have realised that they possess knowledge and skills that may not only be useful to the practice of medical care but also to the practice of other health-related disciplines. Recently nurses themselves are beginning to value their own skills and knowledge and are now much more vocal in decision-making processes, with some holding positions on executive committees (for example, in the development of Primary Care Trusts).

Nurse–doctor interaction today

It is now more than a decade since Stein et al. (1990) revisited the 'game' to evaluate the changes in the intervening years and concluded that nurse–doctor relations had improved. Stein attributed this to the doctors' recognition of their fallibility; reduced public esteem for doctors; increased numbers of female doctors and male nurses together with increased esteem for nurses in their own right rather than as handmaidens. I would argue that if there has been an improvement, it is also as a result of changed nurse education, with the emphasis on more academic training and being prepared for a more autonomous role where the 'handmaiden' role does not play a part. However, as my own reflection indicates, although the relationship may have improved it clearly is not perfect.

It appears that there is still an inequality between the professions despite such close working relationships. Why was I 'not invited to join them (the doctors)?'

Porter (1991) conducted research using nurses and doctors working within ICU in order to study their interactions. He concluded that there were four types of decision-making processes being undertaken:

1 *Unproblematic subordination*: Unquestioning obedience.
2 *Informal covert decision making*: The doctor–nurse game.
3 *Informal overt decision making*: Open involvement of nurses.
4 *Formal overt decision making*: Including the nursing process in decision making.

Whilst model 3 was the most commonly used, he also found that nurse–consultant interactions fell within the nurse–doctor game. This supports the findings of Devine (1978) and is possibly a reflection of the consultants' high status, or the fact that senior members of both professions display attitudes formed when the power gap between nurses and doctors was wider. I recognise the use of model 3 interactions within my story once I had gained access to the meeting, but it does not answer the question of why I was not invited. The findings of Mackay (in Sweet & Norman, 1995) go someway to illuminating my question. Mackay considered the hospital environment to have an effect on the relationship between doctors and nurse; in district hospitals both professions reported an easier, more relaxed atmosphere, whilst in teaching hospitals relations were more formal and competitive, which was often detrimental to working relationships. Whatever the rationale for leaving out the nursing input in the initial discussion regarding Jennie's treatment, I did act upon my strong intuition to join the group; this decision I believe was influenced by my past experiences.

Nurse participation in ethical decision making

Commonly ICU nurses are required to implement procedures (including withdrawal of treatment) when they have not been party to the decision-making process. This may lead to conflict with the doctors and distress for the nurse (Broom, 1991; Erlen & Frost, 1991; Holly & Lyons, 1993; Hustead & Hustead, 1993). It is the nurse who is continually by the bedside with the family and is expected to implement the procedures dictated by the physicians. If doctors take the primary role in decision making, nurses may be left feeling powerless, angry and frustrated (Rodney, 1991).

I can relate to having had these feelings of frustration and of being used as an 'information broker' in past experiences (Holly, 1989). It expends much personal emotion, which inevitably means less than total involvement in caring for the patient. I surmise that these past feelings contributed to my insistence at being present at Jennies discussion; I knew that if I did not go, not only would I be unable to have my technical questions answered, but also important decisions would be made regarding treatment that I (nor any nurse who had looked after Jennie) would have to take part in. Regardless of the nature of the decision, it would only have served to cause distancing of the doctor–nurse relationship. My working relationship with the ICU consultant is based on mutual trust and acknowledgement of differing skills. The lack of invitation to join the group was disappointing but my active participation served to raise his awareness that I was not seeking to undermine his power base. He ultimately has the legal responsibility for any decisions (BMA, 1981) and may well have been feeling some emotional turmoil also; it is, however, difficult to support a colleague in the decision-making process if we are denied input.

Ashley (1974) suggests that medicine and nursing have not developed as a complimentary pair of professional groups sharing common interests and goals; rather they have developed in close proximity, but not sharing common goals and interests. She argues that this in part is due to the paternalistic nature of medicine, as well as its relationship to prestige and power. Grundstein-Amado (1992) concurs with Ashley, whilst Benner (1987) suggests a healthy, functional tension between the two professionals protects the patient from tunnel vision. However, she adds that these tensions need to remain clear of power struggles and status inequity. Whilst it should be possible for two groups of professionals to work together respecting each others skills, including intuitive skills, and knowledge to benefit the patient and avoid moral distress, it could be posited that in attempting to promote the uniqueness of nursing, the profession itself has caused barriers to be built between doctors and nurses. As a result nurses have a tendency to believe that they alone are concerned with the welfare of the patient and according to Henneman (1995) view doctors as the 'enemy', devaluing the therapeutic potential inherent in the doctor–patient association.

In reflecting back on the complex phenomena of the doctor–nurse relationships within the current clinical environment, there seems to be an undercurrent of traditional behaviour by both parties; the doctors did not invite me and I had to request that the nurse in charge relieved me so that I could attend, that is, she did not encourage my participation. In addition, I needed to assert myself within the physicians group before I was acknowledged as being present. However, once I had established myself as a member of the team, they were interested in my contribution and welcomed my perspective. This is an important point to note, as Henneman (1995) suggests that many of the problems related to doctor–nurse relationships are typically blamed on the doctor. She observes that this attitude has resulted in nurses remaining reactive rather than proactive in effecting change in professional collaboration, blocking the therapeutic potential of all involved parties.

Theoretical framing

The incident with the doctors was a very positive one for me and serves to show that it is equally important to be challenged on why something went well, rather than always focusing on negative issues as is often the case in clinical supervision (Rolfe et al., 2001). I did not see my insistence at joining the doctors as a power struggle between the professions but necessary in order to express my caring values. It was important that I did not compromise Jennie, the nursing profession or myself by not committing myself to my beliefs and whilst it would have been less disruptive to the unit had I not attended, I knew that this course of action would have caused me moral distress (Viney, 1996).

Reality perspective framing

It was important for me to share with my supervisor the positive feelings I had experienced because they formed a milestone in my clinical supervision career. I had grown and was striving to work towards my vision of nursing as caring; I felt emancipated and excited by my exploration but at the same time isolated from my colleagues. I had been able, via reflection, to move out of personal emotional entanglement to a position of being able to view Jennie with emotional content but not with over-emotional involvement. I acted, rather than reacted, with emotional distance facilitating my responses (Ramos, 1992) but was left to face the comments of my colleagues who had not had the benefits of clinical supervision.

For the reflective practitioner there is also the challenge of learning about oneself and developing practice whilst investigating theoretical principles. This can be time consuming and exhausting because unless we feel uncomfortable or are forced to look at ourselves, we are unlikely to change, since it is far easier to accept the way things are without questioning (Smyth, 1989). Without the challenge, Jarvis (1992) suggests that 'experts' may face an increased danger of habitualisation compared with novices who are still learning as they go along. Despite the liberating effects of my clinical supervision, it was still challenging to continually question my practice, not least because this meant having to confront the reality that was Jennie's illness.

Following the discussion about Jennie, I was faced by my colleagues' disbelief at what had been proposed but remained very sure that it was the right decision. Whilst understanding the difficulties I felt, my supervisor focused my thoughts on how I was going to deal with them. Using Van Manens' (1977) levels of reflection to illustrate that reflective practice cannot actually transform practice if it is slotted into a culture which is unsympathetic to the ideals, I became aware that the environment is critical to the facilitation of nursing as therapy (see Figure 3.4)

Conway (1998) identified four types of nurse experts: technologists, traditionalists, specialists and humanistic existentialists. Whilst all the experts in Conway's study believed they were reflective, there was little evidence in the traditionalists, some in the technologists and specialists, but mainly of a problem-solving nature. The beliefs that they were reflective enabled them to continue practising as they were and was the antithesis of critical reflexivity. Critical reflective ability was the hallmark of the humanistic existentialist. I struggled with how I might respond to my colleagues' disbelief given that the majority of the practitioners on the unit seemed to be practising as technologists and traditionalists.

It is not the role of a supervisor to prescribe solutions, rather that they should offer one or more examples of specific courses of action that the supervisee can take when considering the options. My overwhelming feeling was one of wanting to share with my colleagues the sense of release I felt within the experience

Technical level	Asking 'how' questions: how do I do something?
Understanding level	Asking 'why' questions: why should I respond in this way rather than that?
Conditions level	What are the underlying norms of practice that determine the way things are? Do these contain desirable work? Can these be changed to facilitate desirable work?

Figure 3.4 *Three levels of reflection; Van Manen (1977)*

and how supervision has provided the space for this to happen, without sounding evangelical. I therefore asked for help in this matter (Bond & Holland, 1998). A number of strategies were discussed:

1 Multi-disciplinary case conference regarding Jennie.
2 Present my reflections at an F grade meeting.
3 Present a teaching session about the process of guided reflection.
4 Seek out nurses with ideals sympathetic to my own.
5 Encourage reflective bedside handovers.
6 Actively ask other nurses how they felt after a tough shift.

I felt comfortable that I could embrace some of these initiatives and reflected that if I were not so keen to increase awareness it could be considered a negative issue surrounding clinical supervision. I agreed to try and action numbers 2–6 before my next clinical supervision. The process of changing a culture was not going to be quick or easy and I was reminded of Charles Handy's 'boiling frogs' (Handy, 1991) and encouraged by the words of Emden:

> Those around you will quickly notice the significance of how you approach your work: a ripple effect becomes evident as others seek to understand and emulate your ideas and practices. (1991: 212)

Problem framing

Already identified problems include:

• clarifying personal beliefs that constitute desirable practice;
• understanding my attitude to Jennie;
• the doctor–nurse relationship;
• nurses role in decision making;
• problems of becoming reflective; and
• changing the cultural norms.

Without guidance I believe I would not have explored all these themes. I had an overriding feeling of euphoria that I wanted others to understand, but only with guidance was I able to discover why I felt like this and use the information in future experiences.

Temporal framing

My supervisor recognised that I had previously brought incidents of 'moral outrage' to my sessions, which had been characterised by energy-draining frustration, anger and a sense of powerlessness as described by Pike (1991). They had occurred when I had been blocked from having input into clinical decision making and had always involved a senior doctor. I reflected that on one occasion I was expected to terminally wean a patient and support the family, having had no input into the decision, causing me to feel frustration and irritation at the lack of collaboration. Through clinical supervision it was possible to explore the situation, realise that research highlighted experiences similar to my own (Pike, 1991; Viney, 1996) and find a way of resolving the conflict I felt. In this instance role-play enabled me to enact the conversation I would have with the doctor involved. Wilkinson (1988) has shown that nurses who are continually affected by moral outrage either protect themselves with coping mechanisms or leave bedside nursing; either way their connection to themselves as therapists is severed. Neither of these options was appropriate for me. A useful technique, taught by my supervisor, is that of thinking upstream (Butterfield, 1990). It highlights the need to anticipate incidents or events prior to them happening and mentally prepare for them and rehearse the options you might use effectively. I could connect with my previous experiences and understood my need to be part of the discussion, not only to prevent moral outrage but also to play my part in developing communications and mutual respect for medical colleagues.

Framing the development of effectiveness

It is not possible to measure effectiveness from one clinical supervision session, although I have described how a previous experience influenced my actions. It is via each practitioner describing their personal and professional growth and the development of therapeutic effectiveness that the impact of clinical supervision can be described for personal use and for managers to understand the importance of it. In order to monitor personal growth and effectiveness, it is necessary to keep accurate notes from each clinical supervision session. These can then be utilised to construct a reflective review enabling the practitioner to:

- look back and see where desirable work was achieved;
- identify where future effort needs to be focused in order to increase effectiveness;
- identify the support needed to achieve effective work;
- incorporate the reflective review with formal appraisal to enable the manager to acknowledge achievements and focus on key areas for development.

(Johns, 1995)

In my development as a reflective practitioner, I realise that I am becoming more questioning and that becoming and remaining a good nurse is relentless work (Davis, 1998). Reflection is becoming central to my practice and a focus for it. The commitment to grow via reflective practice is often painful, but can give moments of insight that lead to great joy, as described in Jennies story. At previous sessions I had brought situations of conflict, problematic areas of practice or difficulties with relatives. This reflection was revelationary for me, since it elicited a feeling of emancipation describing personal movement from domination of emotions to freedom to act according to my true values and beliefs. It did not make an awful scenario better but it did open my eyes to my practice, enabling me to become more therapeutic. It was a high point in my clinical supervision and serves to illustrate how guided reflection enables movement within the 'swampy lowlands' of practice (Schön, 1987).

Conclusion

It is easy for nurses to lose sight of the humanness of their patients. The constant challenge is to balance the science and the art of nursing so that neither dominates the other and that both are seen as complimentary rather than in opposition (Cooper, 1993). Clinical supervision using guided reflective practice has been used in this chapter to illustrate, via a personal story, how this can be achieved and could be applied to any experience within practice. It also highlights the importance of supporting nurses in areas of practice experience that cannot be learnt through academic courses or books. By challenging established practices, supervision may expose rituals, which can be removed to make time for more creative healing nursing. Whilst the theoretical principles of reflection are straightforward, the challenge to become a reflective practitioner is not without hurdles. The description and discussion of the reflection outlined here show the degree of questioning and analysis of practice that is both time consuming and challenging. For the reflective practitioner it is no longer possible to accept anything in practice on face value and the effort required to do this should not be underestimated. It is acknowledged that some nurses may initially feel threatened by this exploration of their practice and its therapeutic value. This highlights the support and guidance required in the supervisory relationship. However, the emancipation of the therapeutic self, along with the experiences of empowerment and enlightenment discovered in the process, more than compensates for the emotional, psychological and physical effort expended.

References

Ashley, J. (1974) *Hospital, Paternalism and the Role of the Nurse*. New York: Teachers College Press.
Benner, P. (1984) *From novice to expert*. Mento Park: Addison Wesley.

Benner, P. (1987) 'A dialogue with excellence – early warning'. *American Journal of Nursing* Dec., 1557–8.

Benner, P. (1991) 'The privacy of caring and the role of experience, narrative and community in clinical ethical expertise'. *Advances in Nursing Science*, **14**: 2, 1–21.

Benner, P., Hooper-Kyriakidis, P. & Stannard, D. (1999) *Clinical Wisdom and Interventions in Critical Care. A thinking in action approach*. Philadelphia: W.B. Saunders.

Benner, P., Tanner, C. & Chelsea, C. (1992) 'From beginner to expert: gaining a differentiated clinical world in critical care nursing'. *Advanced Nursing Science*, **14** (3), 13–28.

Bond, M. & Holland, S. (1998) *Skills of clinical supervision for nurses*. Milton Keynes: Open University Press.

Boykin, A. Schoenhofer, S. (1991) 'Story as a link between nursing practice, ontology and epistemology'. *Image: The Journal of Nursing Scholarship*, **23** (4), 245–8.

British Medical Association (1981) *The Handbook of Medical Ethics*. London: British Medical Association.

Brookfield, S. (1987) *Developing critical thinkers*. Milton Keynes: Open University Press.

Broom, C. (1991) 'Conflict resolution strategies Dimensions'. *Critical Care Nursing,* **10**: 6, 354–64.

Butterfield, P. (1990) 'Thinking Upstream: nurturing a conceptual understanding of the societal context of health behaviour'. *Advanced Nursing Science*, **12** (2), 1–8.

Butterworth, A. & Faugier, J. (1994) *Clinical Supervision and Mentorship in Nursing*. London: Chapman Hall.

Carper, B. (1978) 'Fundamental patterns of knowing in nursing'. *Advances in Nursing Science,* **1** (1), 13–23.

Conway, J. (1998) 'Evolution of the species "expert nurse". An examination of the practical knowledge held by expert nurses'. *Journal of Clinical Nursing*, **7**: 1, 75–82.

Cooper, M. (1993) 'The intersection of technology of care in the ICU'. *Advanced Nursing Science*, **15** (3), 23–32.

Davis, M. (1998) 'The rocky road to reflection' in Johns, C. & Freshwater, D. (eds) *Transforming Nursing Through Reflective Practice*, Oxford: Blackwell Scientific. Ch. 17.

Devine, B. (1978) 'Nurse-physician interaction: Status and social structure within two hospital wards'. *Journal of Advanced Nursing*, **2**: 3, 278–95.

Erlen, J. & Frost, B. (1991) 'Nurses' perceptions of powerlessness in influencing ethical decisions'. *Western Journal of Nursing Research*, **13**: 3, 397–407.

Fay, B. (1987) *Critical Social Science*. Cambridge: Polity Press.

Frank, A.W. (2000) 'The standpoint of storyteller'. *Qualitative Health Research*, **10**: 3, 354–65.

Freshwater, D. (1998) 'Transforming Nursing through Reflective Practice'. Unpublished PhD Thesis. University of Nottingham.

Grundstein-Armado, R. (1992) 'Differences in ethical decision making processes among doctors and nurses'. *Journal of Advanced Nursing*, **17**: 2, 129–37.

Handy, C. (1991) *The age of unreason,* 2nd edn. London: Century Business.

Henneman, E. (1995) 'Nurse-physician collaboration: a post structuralist view'. *Journal of Advanced Nursing*, **22**: 2, 359–63.

Holly, C. (1989) 'Critical care nurses' participation in ethical decision-making'. *Journal of New York State Nursing Association*, **20**: 4, 9–12.

Holly, C. & Lyons, M. (1993) 'Increasing your decision-making role in ethical situations'. *Dimensions in Critical Care*, **12**: 5, 264–71.

Hustead, J. & Hustead, G. (1993) 'Personal and interpersonal values in bioethical decision making'. *Journal of Health Care Practice,* **5**, 59–65.

Jarvis, P. (1992) 'Reflective Practice and Nursing'. *Nurse Education Today*, **12**: 3, 174–81.

Johns, C. (1993) 'On becoming effective in ethical action'. *Journal of Clinical Nursing*, **32**: 5, 307–312.

Johns, C. (1995) 'The value of reflective practice'. *Journal of Clinical Nursing*, 4 (1), 23–30.

Johns, C. (1997) 'Reflective practice and clinical supervision – Part II Guiding learning through reflection to structure the supervision "space"'. *European Nurse*, 2 (3), 192–204.

Johns, C. (1998) 'Opening the doors of perception' in Johns, C. & Freshwater, D. (eds) *Transforming Nursing Through Reflective Practice*. Oxford: Blackwell Scientific. Ch. 1.

Keddy, B., Gillis, M., Jacobs, P., Burton, H. & Rogers, M. (1986) 'The doctor–nurse relationship: an historical perspective'. *Journal of Advanced Nursing*, 11: 6, 745–53.

Marks-Maran, D. & Rose, P. (1997) *Reconstructing Nursing: beyond art and science*. London: Balliere Tindall.

May, C. (1991) 'Affective neutrality and involvement in nurse patient relationships: perceptions of appropriate behaviour amongst nurses in acute medical and surgical wards'. *Journal of Advanced Nursing*, 16: 5, 552–8.

Menzies, I.E.P. (1988) *Containing Anxiety in Institutions: selected essays*. London: Free Association Books.

Mishler, E.G. (1986) 'The analysis of interview-narratives'. in Sarbin, T. (ed.) *Narrative Psychology: the storied nature of human conduct.*. New York: Praeger. p. 111–25.

Morse, J. (1991) 'Negotiating commitment and involvement in the nurse–patient relationship'. *Journal of Advanced Nursing*, 16: 4, 455–68.

Morse, J., Bottoroff, J., Anderson, G., O'Brien, B. & Solberg, S. (1992) 'Beyond empathy: expanding expressions of caring'. *Journal of Advanced Nursing*, 17: 7, 809–821.

Munhall, P. (1994) *Revisioning Phenomenology. Nursing and Health Science Research*. New York: National League for Nurses.

NHS Management Executive (1993) *A Vision for the Future: the nursing, midwifery and health visiting contribution to health care*. Department of Health. London: HMSO.

Pike, A. (1991) 'Moral outrage and moral discourse in nurse physician collaboration'. *Journal of Professional Nursing*, 7 (6), 351–63.

Porter, S. (1991) 'A participant observation study of power relations between nurses and doctors in a general hospital'. *Journal of Advanced Nursing*, 16: 6, 728–35.

Ramos, M. (1992) 'The nurse–patient relationship: theme and variations'. *Journal of Advanced Nursing*, 17: 4, 496–506.

Ray, M. (1987) 'Technological caring: a new model in critical care'. *Dimensions in Critical Care Nursing*, 6: 3, 169–73.

Rodney, P. (1991) 'Dealing with ethical problems. An ethical decision-making model for critical care nurses'. *Canadian Critical Care Nursing*, 8: 1, 8–10.

Rolfe, G., Freshwater, D. & Jasper, M. (2001) *Critical Reflection for Nurses and the Helping Professions*. Basingstoke: Palgrave.

Schön, D. (1987) *Educating the Reflective Practitioner*. San Francisco: Jossey Bass.

Smyth, J. (1989) 'Developing and sustaining critical reflection in teacher education'. *Journal of Teacher Education*, 40 (2), 2–9.

Stein, L. (1978) 'The doctor–nurse game' in Dingwall, R. & McIntosh, J. (eds) *Reading in the Sociology of Nursing*. Edinburgh: Churchill Livingstone. Ch. 7.

Stein, L., Watts, D. & Howell, T. (1990) 'The doctor–nurse game revisited'. *New England Journal of Medicine*, 322 (8), 546–9.

Sweet, S. & Norman, I. (1995) 'The nurse–doctor relationship: a selective literature review'. *Journal of Advanced Nursing*, 22: 1, 165–70.

United Kingdom Central Council (1996) *Position statement on clinical supervision for nursing and health visiting*. London: United Kingdom Central Council for Nursing, Midwifery and Health Visiting.

Van Manen, M. (1977) 'Linking ways of knowing with ways of being'. *Curriculum Inquiry*, 6: 3, 205–228.

Vezeau, T. (1994) 'Narrative inquiry in nursing' in Chinn, P. & Watson, J. (eds) *Art and Aesthetics in Nursing.* New York: National League for Nursing. Ch. 3.

Viney, C. (1996) 'A phenomenological study of ethical decision making among senior intensive care doctors and nurses concerning with withdrawal of treatment'. *Nursing in Critical Care,* **1** (4), 182–7.

Watson, J. (1988a) 'New dimensions of human caring theory'. *Nursing Science Quarterly,* **9** (4), 175–81.

Watson, J. (1988b) *Nursing: Human science and human care. A theory of nursing.* New York: National League for Nurses.

Wilkinson, J. (1988) 'Moral experience in nursing practice: experience and effect'. *Nursing Forum,* **23**: 1, 16–19.

Wright, S. (1985) 'New nurses: new boundaries'. *Nursing Practice,* **1** (1), 32–9.

Younger, T. (1990) 'Literary works as a mode of knowing'. *Image: The Journal of Nursing Scholarship,* **22** (1), 39–43.

4 The Role of the Internal Supervisor in Developing Therapeutic Nursing

Gillian Todd

This chapter, based on a research project, is divided into three parts; the introduction sets the scene, examining the theoretical foundations of reflexivity in relation to the self. Theoretical foundations of reflexive case study, which was used to investigate the therapeutic use of the self in the role of clinical supervisor, are introduced alongside the ontological considerations and the epistemological roots that informed the inquiry. As reflexive case study is about contextualizing practice, the concept of the self within a postmodernist perspective is explored and its influences on qualitative methodology scrutinized.

In the second part a series of case vignettes from clinical practice and reflexive case studies explore the process of developing the self as a therapeutic tool within a cognitive behavioural framework. This part presents the intrinsic dynamics of developing insight and awareness of the internal supervisor as a therapeutic tool from reflection-on-action to reflection-in-action. The construct of the self is viewed from a cognitive behavioural perspective. Evidence from clinical practice is presented with the aim of enabling the reader to understand complex ideas and how conclusions were arrived at.

In part three the impact that the process of reflection-in-action has upon both the practitioner and on patient outcomes are discussed. The concluding discussion reflects on the evidence derived from the reflexive case studies, which suggests that the practitioner, in developing awareness of the self from reflection-on-action to reflection-in-action, had a direct influence on patient outcomes.

Theoretical foundations

In this section I outline the theoretical foundations of a reflexive case study that explored the questions: What is the process in developing my self-reflective internal supervisor in-action? What are the cognitive and behavioural processes in the development of the participants internal supervisor from reflection-on-action to reflection-in-action? In what ways does the operation of the internal supervisor-in-action bring changes and evidence into clinical practice?

Casement (1985) first conceptualised the 'internal supervisor'. In the context of clinical supervision, the development of the internal supervisor is seen as an advanced part of the reflective process (Bond & Holland, 1998). The supervisee progressively moves from a focus of reflection-on-action within clinical supervision that provides a forum for developing self-awareness and insight into their clinical practice. The internal supervisor is born when the supervisee develops the capacity for spontaneous reflection-in-action; moving from retrospective reflection to an awareness of one's thoughts and reactions to any given situation in the moment. The internal supervisor is the inner voice that provides an objective perspective of a situation whilst in parallel questioning subjectivity.

Schön (1983) believes the practitioner becomes a researcher in the practice context when reflecting-in-action through reframing problematic situations, then converting new knowledge into behaviour change. The role of researcher/practitioner is central to reflexive research methodology. The researcher/practitioner becomes participant observer in reflectively exploring their practice (Rolfe, 1997). I, as researcher/practitioner, will reflectively explore my practice as clinical supervisor, drawing upon my subjective data through reflection-on-action in combination with external data from interviews and reflective journals.

I begin with the premise that studying the development of the internal supervisor through reflexive practice in clinical supervision evolved as a result of my own value system, history and interest. My situation as a researcher/practitioner is inseparable from many other traditions in which I am engaged, such as my knowledge and experiences as a cognitive therapist and a nurse. Thus the subsequent chapter and the interpretations that follow are influenced by what precedes these situations through comparison to previous knowledge and experience. As Koch states, 'the situation of the researcher can never be separated from the ongoing traditions in which she is engaged' (1998: 887). Hence I embarked upon this research study believing that neither the researcher nor the participant can assume a privileged position in the interpretation of knowledge, as pre-understandings brought to the research need to be explored within a collaborative process. A question then arises: Is it possible to study the participant without studying myself within that process? And is that process static in taking snapshots, or a continuous marriage of self-awareness and self-critique?

Walters's, in analysing human condition, notes that 'people are in and of the world, rather than subjects in a world of objects' (1995: 793). Hence what is reality at one point in time might not be in a different context. The only person who can mediate and articulate this dynamic reality is the individual themselves, that is to say that the individual is the expert on themselves – this includes the nurse reflecting and developing their practice.

In the theory of cognitive therapy as described by Beck et al. (1979), the individual is also considered to be the experts on themselves. The process of therapy involves collaboratively entering into the individual's worldview whilst simultaneously developing an awareness of your own reactions, attitudes and beliefs that influence interpretations as a therapist. The process of reflexivity stimulates critical reflection in looking inwards on ourselves, making the unconscious conscious in bringing a new awareness to the internal experience. King, in conceptualising how we use the therapeutic self as researcher, states: 'the self is viewed not as static, but rather as a multiplicity of complex, often contradictory, fragmented or plural identities. In such the self is always in flux' (1996: 175). Given that the self is a fluid concept that moulds and changes in different contexts, it is appropriate to re-examine the self (whether nurse, patient or therapist) as researcher within a social constructionalist epistemology.

Rolfe (1997), viewing the broader context of nursing practice, suggests that to be an effective practitioner the nurse must look beyond the scientific paradigm and theory into a wider epistemological base that can provide a deeper understanding of practice. It could be argued that unless the epistemological base for reflection is understood it would become nothing more than a technique that applies theory to practice (Freshwater, 1998). Given that reflexive case study is about narrative (in that I act as participant observer of my own practice, narrating the story I observe), the epistemological basis of this chapter is embedded within the constuctionalist epistemology. Postmodernism also has some affiliation with constructivist epistemology as the belief systems are evaluated in terms of their current feasibility in particular contexts. Safran & Muran (2000) referred to this process as developing an awareness of one's own construction of reality as it takes place. There is an opposition to the objectivist epistemology that is congruent with modernism. Adopting a modernist perspective in reflexive research methodology, the researcher would be a scientist-practitioner, who in the role of researcher would be always objective, unbiased and free from value-laden assumptions, beliefs and prejudices. This stance is incongruent with that of a reflexivity in which the self as researcher adopts the view that there is no objective datum, no single truth or reality. Lyddon & Weill (1997), in discussing truth and reality within a postmodern view, suggest that reality is socially constructed, inhabited by people rather than having been given and as such may change and vary in time and context across cultures. Hence within the context of reflexivity, reflections of memories, thoughts, beliefs and experiences of the researcher/ practitioner and the participant are understood within the point in time they occur through reflection-in and on-action and are contingent upon the symbolic resources of the culture (Potter, 1996). Safran & Muran (2000) refer to this concept as mindfulness, a practice that involves developing awareness in the moment through self-exploration whilst maintaining a non-judgemental stance.

If reflexive research methodology is a self-reflexive inquiry within a constructionist epistemology, it is important to understand the concept of the self from a postmodern perspective. In 1934, Mead (cited in King, 1996: 175) described the reflexive self as 'the turning back of the experience of the individual upon her or himself'. The relationship between reflexivity and the self is complex, as the self as researcher enters into an intricate web with endless spiralling dynamics and perceptions (King, 1996). The self becomes a socially constructed concept that is dynamic and fluid, continually constructed and reconstructed in a range of social and cultural contexts over time (Clark, 1997). Sullivan, 1953 (cited in Safran & Muran, 2000), discusses how reflected appraisals of others determine how we experience personal characteristics belonging to the self which are most valued by others. Both positive and negative characteristics become personified as part of the self as 'good me' or 'bad me'. For example, Margaret, a 51-year-old university lecturer, was referred for a course of cognitive therapy for depression. In understanding her vulnerability to depression, the theme of failure was central to relapses. As a child academic, excellence was valued, whilst her artistic talents were discounted as unimportant; if she attained top marks praise was given and anything less than perfection resulted in criticism. Margaret developed the belief that 'good me' equated to perfection and 'bad me' meant failure.

As an adult when faced with situations where Margaret's high standards were not met, she would see herself as bad and a failure; this would escalate into a vicious cycle of depression. Developing both positive and negative beliefs about the self influence the way in which the individual relates to their inner and outer worlds; this has been referred to as a relational matrix by which people behave in such a way that maintains their relatedness to others (Safran & Muran, 2000).

The researcher/practitioner

As a participant observer of my own practice, my self will become: self as narrative and dialogue; self as self theory; self as an evolving process; self as possible selves; self as community; and self as therapeutic. My self consists of multiple self-states that are compatible with one another to varying degrees. Depending on the relational context, multifarious self-states become dominant at distinctive times, just as a chameleon changes its appearance in adapting to different environments. Safran and Muran suggest that 'each individual experiences a perpetual cycle between different self states, which in turn evoke complimentary self state in the other' (2000: 67). They criticise the view that holding a unitary perception of the self is nothing more than an illusion that is socially and historically constructed. As a researcher/practitioner I become an integral part of my inquiry to identify the processes that are involved in developing and operationalising my internal supervisor whilst simultaneously observing the development and interaction of the supervisee's internal supervisor through reflexivity (Casement, 1985).

One criticism of postmodernism in the context of reflexivity is that in exploring a person's reality in how they make sense of the world, there is no place to explore the cognitive processes themselves in discovering the meaning of cognition. Gergen & Gergen (1991) explain:

> ... by means of critical reflection and an examination and exploration of the research process from different positions, the aim of trying to use our reflexivity is to move us outward to achieve an expansion of understanding. (Cited in King 1996: 176)

This relational approach is in sharp contrast to an introspective one, because it then becomes possible to transcend the very parameters in which the research is being carried out.

As such reflexive research is an ideal methodology (based on a constructionalist epistemology) for studying myself in relation to others as storytellers, theory generators and active participants in a collaborative inquiry, which aims to describe the process and dynamics of the internal supervisor.

The development of the dynamic internal supervisor

Clinical supervision provides a platform in which insight can be gained through the process of reflection-on-action (Johns & Freshwater, 1998). However, engaging in nostalgic reflections about elements of practice experience is not adequate in facilitating the development of awareness in one's immediate experiences, that is, reflection-in-action.

Safran & Muran (2000) argue that whilst retrospective reflection about aspects of one's experiences can play an important role in the change process, it is not sufficient in and of itself. It is only through the immediate awareness of experiences that new possibilities emerge. But how do you move from retrospective reflection to developing awareness in the moment through reflection-in-action? Are they mutually exclusive or is the relationship between both dimensions of reflection reciprocal?

Central to reflection is the development of the reflexive internal supervisor in-action. Within a cognitive behavioural framework the dynamics of the self are understood from Beck et al.'s (1979) theory, based on the premise that repeated occurrences of negative early experience lead to the formation of negative self-schemata. The schema is the cognitive structure and within Beck's theory the content of the schema, that is on a belief and assumption level, is what is important. Beliefs are self-relevant, unconditional in nature and core constructs; for example, 'I'm a failure', 'I'm unlovable'. They are viewed as facts about perception of oneself and how the world and other people are viewed. Assumptions are conditional and tend to be 'if … then' propositions, for example, 'If I put others needs first then they will approve of me'. When a person is faced with a critical incident depending on the personal value and specific meaning that the individual places on the situation, it is thought that negative self-schemata (cognitive vulnerability) will be activated, which generates specific negative automatic thoughts (NAT's). NAT's lead to changes in emotions that feedback into accentuating patterns of negative thinking, which impact on physical and behavioural reactions and if unchallenged lead to reinforcing a negative view of self.

Case example

Michaela is a 19-year-old student with bulimia nervosa. She was teased at school because of her weight problem; this made her decide to diet. As she became thinner she noticed her popularity increase amongst her peers. A starvation diet lead to binge eating and in fear of her gaining weight Michaela would engage in compensatory behaviour such as self-induced vomiting and laxative use. Working together we formulated an understanding of Michaela's self within a cognitive behavioural framework that is illustrated in Figure 4.1.

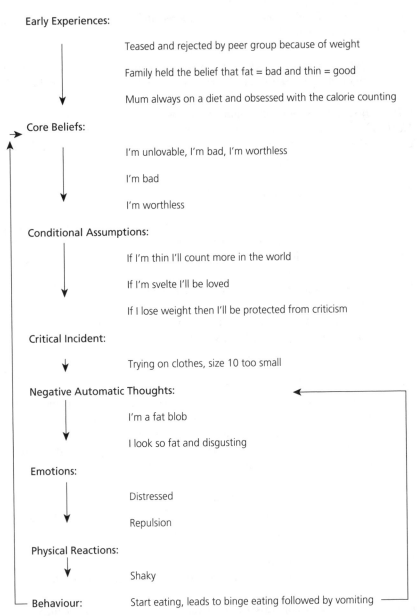

Figure 4.1   *Michaela: a cognitive formulation (adapted from Beck et al.'s*
Cognitive Model, 1979)

Within a cognitive behavioural construct of the self, the self-concept can change from one situation to another, mediated by an individual's cognitive vulnerability. This is illustrated through an extract from a clinical supervision session with Mark, who works as a community psychiatric nurse in elderly care. During clinical supervision he described feeling stressed and losing interest in his

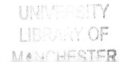

work; through reflection-on-action we explored this situation, further entering into a Socratic dialogue:

Mark: I've had a terrible week. I'm stressed all the time. Yesterday in the referral meeting I was given three new assessments to complete and don't feel able to cope.

CS: It sounds like you're completely overwhelmed.

Mark: Yes, I am, I'm counting my time away until retirement.

CS: You're really having a hard time. Would it be helpful for us to try and understand your distress?

Mark: Yes.

CS: When you were feeling overwhelmed, what was running through your mind?

Mark: I can't take it anymore, the work never ends; these patients need to be seen, and as usual it's all down to me.

CS: What was it that made you think that it was all down to you to do the work?

Mark: Well, it's got to be done and if others don't volunteer then I've got to make it right.

CS: So is it that you feel responsible for other people in the team and try and make everything run smoothly even though it makes you feel bad?

Mark: Yes, that's exactly right.

CS: What do you think the advantages and disadvantages are of trying to make everything all right?

Mark: The advantages are those patients are seen. People like me and it helps keep the peace. The disadvantages are that I'm putting unrealistic pressures on myself and consequently stressed out. I'm less thorough with my work and can be irritable with patients. I'm a grumpy and take it out on my family. Worse of I lost respect from my colleagues and can be taken for granted.

CS: Weighing up the balance, what do you think?

Mark: I'm putting others first 100 per cent of the time; I'm neglecting my own needs and in doing so compromise my professionalism.

CS: How can you get out of this trap?

Mark: I need to learn to say no more often.

CS: What plan do we need to develop to put these ideas into practice?

Through developing a cognitive behavioural construct of Mark's self-perception in this situation allowed him to gain insight into possible reasons that maintained his feelings of stress. Intellectually knowing the benefits of being assertive in a work situation doesn't necessarily influence behavioural change when faced with a similar situation in the future. The clinical supervision session can provide a laboratory in which to explore and experiment with ideas such as self-awareness and skill development, but how can these concepts be transferred into new situations? One way is through developing the internal supervisor in-action that aims to narrow the gap between the experiential and rational mind (Epstein, 1998). It was this gap that I proposed to explore within the current research study.

Process

The method of data collection used throughout my study was that of reflection-on-action through clinical supervision. I, (the researcher/practitioner) and participant Emma, maintained a reflective journal for the duration of the research, documenting our reflection-on-action in relation to the utilisation of the internal supervisor in-action. In addition notes were taken during the clinical supervision sessions and two sessions were audio-taped (session three and session six) for the raw data. The tapes were then transcribed to enable reflection on the development of the internal supervisor. Pre and post research interviews were conducted with the participant to facilitate reflection on the research process, feedback and checking data analysis. Six key themes were identified relating to the process of developing the internal supervisor (see Figure 4.2 for summary).

Before elaborating on the themes identified in developing the internal supervisor, my reflections on the process of being as researcher/practitioner itself will be shared. Writing this chapter has involved experiencing my internal world in different ways and this at times has felt uncomfortable, often ending in procrastination. As a novice clinical supervisor I organised group supervision for ward nurses. At first no one engaged in the process. From a technical perspective I was doing it right, but it wasn't working. I tracked my own reactions in this situation and noticed that I was feeling frustration towards the participants. I thought, 'I'm wasting my time here, sit it out, you've only four groups left to go.' I was not using myself in a therapeutic way in utilising my internal supervisor to question my reactions in moving towards developing a therapeutic alliance.

Theme	Description of the theme
1	Collaborative empiricism In developing the internal supervisor
2	Selecting the clinical supervisor to facilitate the development of the internal supervisor
3	Socialisation into the theoretical model of reflexivity in conceptualising the internal supervisor
4	Barriers to reflexivity: cognitive processes that effect the internal supervisor
5	Enhancing the internal supervisor: strategies that promote reflexivity
6	The internal supervisor in developing the researcher as participant self-observer

Figure 4.2 *Summary of the process in developing the internal supervisor*

As a consequence of this reflection-on-action I asked the next group to voice their fears around the process of change. As a result of researching my own practice, I learnt that before embarking on the process of developing the dynamics of the internal supervisor, the paradox of change needs to be addressed. Safran & Muran observe that 'the desire to change is the source of pain' (2000: 67) that involves what they refer to as an act of surrender. In developing the internal supervisor, it is important to become aware of your beliefs, cognitive biases and reactions in the moment whether you are in many of the roles that you occupy. Through cultivating awareness and self-acceptance, the therapeutic alliance is developed, thus making it safe for the patient or the supervisors to have faith in changing. Hilliard et al. (2000) proposed a theory that linked the patient's and therapist's interpersonal histories in exploring the processes that occurred during therapy. They noticed the impact of the therapist's own interpersonal history on the therapeutic work. Within postmodern philosophy, the self is perceived as an illusion that adapts and changes from one situation to the next, where the self is inseparable from your experiences. Becoming aware of and acknowledging your own subjectivity opens the doors to possibilities and change. This point is illustrated through an extract from my reflective diary:

> As a child emotion was rarely expressed. When tears were shed embarrassment and apologies would quickly follow, or alternatively comfort would be shown by saying cheer up, or come on now it's not so bad, you've no reason to behave like that. I developed the belief if you expressed emotions then you are weak.

Consequently, when working as a therapist, if a patient expressed emotion I immediately felt uncomfortable. My own discomfort with emotion made it difficult for me to accept emotion experienced by others, which subsequently inhibited the therapeutic alliance. In accepting this as an issue I was able to formulate this from a cognitive behavioural framework, enabling me to acknowledge my fears and question them. Reflection-on-action provides an opportunity to develop a good therapeutic alliance where healing can potentially take place and a platform for developing the internal supervisor in-action can be built.

Discussion of the themes arising from the work

Theme 1: Collaborative empiricism in developing the internal supervisor

Contemporary nursing, and indeed healthcare, readily refers to the term 'collaboration' that is defined by Allen (1993) as 'working jointly' and forms the basis of many recent health policies. Within the context of an evolving therapeutic alliance the interpretation of collaboration is more complex. As Greenberger comments, 'The collaborative relationship can be thought of as two people providing different areas of expertise in pursuit of a common goal' (1992: 141). Whether you occupy the role of nurse, therapist, supervisor or supervisee entering into a relationship that is both collaborative and empirical in exploring the evidence, is fundamental to the process of change. In developing a truly collaborative relationship Emma, an intensive care nurse, and I, needed to share an understanding of our working relationship in order to develop internal harmony and reduce the conflict between the dialogues.

Zuroff et al. (2000) suggest that in parallel to the treatment process there is a need to alert the patient to the alliance issues; when collaboration breaks down the process of working through these ruptures serve to strengthen the alliance and hence produce a better outcome. Although this knowledge refers to clinical practice, parallels can be seen within the supervisory relationship where the objective is to help the supervisee develop skills as an effective reflective practitioner who, through the internal supervisor, can bring evidence into clinical practice through critical reflexivity. Within this reflexive case study of Emma as a supervisee and of myself as a clinical supervisor, our common goal in researching our own practice was to develop the internal supervisor through refection-on-action in clinical supervision and to explore the circular processes that facilitate reflection-in-action.

Critical to clinical supervision and indeed any therapeutic alliance (including the nurse–patient relationship) is the therapeutic relationship. Warmth, genuineness and accurate empathy (Rogers, 1951) facilitate the supervisory process along with trust, rapport and collaboration as the hallmarks of the interaction between supervisor and supervisee (Beck et al., 1979; Butterworth, 1994). Martin et al. (2000), in conducting a meta-analysis of studies measuring the impact of the therapeutic alliance, concluded that collaboration is essential for the therapeutic alliance that is predictive of positive outcomes. The process of developing a collaborative relationship through reflexivity was identified, as were potential barriers that are illustrated in Figure 4.3.

An environmental barrier to collaboration that precluded change was identified; in Emma's clinical setting a hierarchical cascading system of clinical supervision was implemented. Emma remarked, 'It's like Big Brother is watching you.' She perceived clinical supervision as secretive and elitist, which reinforced her belief that the managers were planning to catch you out. In light of her suspicions, Emma held conflicting views about the perceived usefulness of clinical supervision, one that idealised clinical supervision as a panacea, the other which denigrated it, thus creating cognitive dissonance. In exploring this dichotomy the conflicting views were also evident in the literature. In *A Vision for the Future* (Department of Health, 1993) clinical supervision is advocated as an enabling, empowering process that helps nurses develop skills of self-evaluation and reflective analysis. This paper lacked clarity, thus leaving the implementation of clinical supervision open to misinterpretation. For example: Johns (1993); Northcott (1996); and Farrington (1998), who held a managerial agenda that proposed linking clinical supervision to an appraisal system. Cutliffe and Proctor (1998a) surmise that there are five main reasons for the resistance to clinical supervision: it is viewed as a managerial tool; it is seen as a form of personal therapy; there is a lack of clarity about the purpose; there is resistance to change; and the culture of discomfort around emotional expression.

In exploring this barrier through Socratic questioning in the context of collaborative empiricism, Emma and I dismantled the hierarchy in becoming partners in creating a culture of honesty and openness in giving constructive feedback (Hawkins & Shohet, 1989).

Barriers to collaboration

1 The supervisee may lack the necessary skills to collaborate.
2 The supervisee may lack the skill to be collaborative.
3 Environmental stresses may be a preclusion to change.
4 The supervisee's ideas and beliefs about failure in clinical supervision, contributing to non-collaboration.
5 The supervisee's beliefs and ideas about changing and their effects on others as a preclusion to compliance.
6 Supervisee's fear of changing into the new self.
7 The supervisor's and supervisee's dysfunctional beliefs might be harmoniously blended.
8 Poor socialisation into clinical supervision and reflexive case study.
9 Poor timing of interventions can lead to non-compliance in clinical supervision.
10 The supervisee may lack motivation.
11 The supervisee's rigidity may foil compliance.
12 The goals of clinical supervision may be unrealistic, unstated and vague, with no clear agreement between supervisor and supervisee.
13 The supervisor and supervisee may be frustrated because of lack of progress in clinical supervision.

Figure 4.3   *Barriers to reflection-on-action in clinical supervision (adapted from the work of Beck et al., 1990,* Cognitive Therapy of Personality Disorders, *Ch. 4)*

In summary, collaborative empiricism is fundamental in establishing and maintaining a therapeutic alliance, which itself is a central interpersonal process in developing awareness of the multiplicity of the self within divergent contexts. Clinical supervision provides a culture where the internal supervisor, whilst reflecting-in-action, can recognise barriers to collaboration formulated against a cognitive behaviour framework.

Theme 2: Selecting the clinical supervisor to facilitate the development of the internal supervisor

Emma and I questioned the advantages and disadvantages of selecting a supervisor versus being allocated a supervisor. This led to further exploration regarding the personal attributes that a clinical supervisor would need to possess in order to help the supervisee develop their internal supervisor. Two perspectives were taken: the first being the selection of myself as clinical supervisor; the second was the importance of preparing to be a supervisee in developing reflection-in-action.

Figure 4.4 illustrates the attributes of a good clinical supervisor as depicted in the literature.

The literature suggests personal attributes and characteristics determine the selection of the clinical supervisor. In every case the supervisor is portrayed idealistically with a perfect and flawless persona. The depiction of the clinical supervisor as having exemplary standards is illusory, which provides ammunition for the sceptics in denigrating clinical supervision as ineffective in producing positive change in the practitioner. Viewing the qualities of a clinical supervisor in

Summary of key points

1 • Good and relevant knowledge base demonstrated.
  • Good teaching and supervisory skills.
  • Good relationship skills.
  • Values the supervisee as an individual.
  • Demonstrates effort and puts themselves out.
  (Fowler, 1995)

2 • Experience of personal and professional reflection.
  • Functions at a high level.
  • Competent in a wide range of skills, activities and therapeutic modalities.
  • Ability to order and to analyse critically.
  • Skilled in exploring research and scholarship of a personal and academic nature.
  • Competent in dealing with the feelings of the supervisor and supervisee.
  (Chambers, 1995)

3 • Good interpersonal skills.
  • Resource person.
  • Encouraging.
  • To have a benevolent presence.
  • Demonstrates empathy.
  • Promotes good patient care.
  • Giver of positive reinforcement.
  • Confident persona.
  • Good role model.
  • Empowers the supervisee.
  • Supports the supervisee.
  • Develops the supervisee.
  • Performing the multiple roles of effective communicator, teacher, facilitator, advisor, change agent, researcher and as a promoter of high clinical standards.
  (Friedman and Marr, 1995)

4 • Listening skills.
  • Questioning skills.
  • Mirroring and reflecting skills.
  • To respect the privileged position of being chosen as a supervisor.
  (Devine, 1995)

5 • Enable and develop the practitioner.
  • Supervisors in supervision themselves.
  • Adopt a non-judgmental approach.
  • A facilitator of professional development and learning.
  • Empathic.
  • Sound clinical knowledge and competence (not necessarily of the supervisor's discipline).
  • Stress management skills.
  • Empowerer and supervisee led.
(Stoke and McClarey, 1995)

6 • Assessing.
  • Being organised.
  • Being approachable.
  • Giving feedback.

Continued

- Giving responsibility.
- Having realistic expectations.
(Munroe, 1998)

7 Control is with the supervisee.
- Increase the supervisees self-confidence, self-esteem and assertiveness skills.
- Provide time for reflection upon experiences.
- Support.
- To help cope with the fear of being not seen to cope.
- Adequately trained.
(White et al., 1998)

8 • Qualities of the supervisor depend upon adequate training of the supervisee.
- Facilitator of reflective practice.
- Collaboration, the sharing of aims, ground rules, values and terms.
- Self awareness.
- Interpersonal and intrapersonal skills.
- Ability to be a 'comrade'.
(Cutcliffe and Proctor, 1998b)

Figure 4.4   *A literature review summarising the important attributes of a clinical supervisor*

both static and dichotomous dimensions prevents seeing shades of grey, arguably the dimensions that help us to understand the components of the process in selecting the supervisor in developing the reflexive internal supervisor. If clinical supervision is collaborative in sharing with the supervisee a voice of feeling through the creation of language, then the relationship between the supervisee and supervisor needs to be examined in identifying blocks to the supervisory process (Greenwald & Young, 1998). How are the beliefs of the supervisor and supervisee affecting the clinical supervision process, and are their parallels in clinical practice? If the supervisor is helping the supervisee to develop their internal supervisor, who is helping the supervisor develop their internal supervisor, and is this achieved through a parallel process?

The modelling of high-quality supervision influences the style of the supervisee, gradually progressing in to the role of supervisor (Paolo, 1998). A further dimension is the concept that the clinical supervisor never becomes an expert in their role, that is, a continuous evolving process of learning and exploration. Just as we learn from our patients who enable us to grow and develop as skilled practitioners, we can learn from our supervisees (Casement, 1985).

Liese and Alford (1998) believe that central to the supervisory process is the clinical supervisor maintaining confident humility in the search for good supervision. They comment that this will aid the supervision by showing respect for the supervisee's skills and knowledge, which helps to build confidence. Displaying a function as a coping model, publicly recognising their limitations and weaknesses whilst simultaneously striving to be competent, benefits as their clinical supervisory experience broadens.

A combination of positive characteristics, awareness of the components of the process of supervision, and the ability to be collaborative provides the foundations in facilitating the development of the internal supervisor. In entering into the process of reflexivity, the supervisor needs to be in clinical supervision themselves to reflect-on-action in developing and in objectively maintaining their internal supervisor (Titchen & Binnie, 1995).

Theme 3: Socialisation into the theoretical model of reflexivity in developing the internal supervisor

I was left with a dilemma in relation to my work with Emma and the notion of collaborative research, namely: how can you understand a situation unless you have the theoretical knowledge in which to base those experiences? The dilemma of how much of the research protocol I should share with Emma and what would be the most effective strategy in helping her to develop a shared conceptualisation of the internal supervisor. I carefully considered the advantages and disadvantages of full disclosure verses partial ethically correct disclosure. I eventually decided upon full disclosure: Figure 4.5 illustrates the process of reaching this decision.

The research protocol, literature about reflexive case study (Rolfe, 1998) and information on keeping a reflective journal were also presented to Emma (Heath, 1998; Johns, 1995). In becoming a researcher of my practice through reflecting on the parallel process in the research, it was equally important for Emma to research her own practice in facilitating the development of her internal supervisor. How could she have understood what was required of her unless she had equal access to relevant knowledge?

Theme 4: Barriers to reflexivity: cognitive processes that effect the internal supervisor

It is easy to assume that the dynamic internal supervisor who is self-aware always recognises shifting self-states within the perspective of multiple selves bringing in the rational mind to challenge negative attitudes and reactions. Is it possible to rely upon the internal supervisor to bring new perspectives to situations, and would not trusting the internal supervisor add up to not trusting oneself? The process of reflexive case study methodology provided an understanding of what influenced an individual to ignore their internal supervisor. I questioned what the processes were involved in relating to the reflexive internal supervisor in certain events. I hypothesised about reasons that explained why our internal supervisors are blocked in some situations. One explanation could be distortions in how we process information including, for example, thinking and learning styles.

Cognitive distortions as described by Beck et al. (1979) and Burns (1981) provide a negative way of interpreting information that questions the value of the self and give rise to emotional distress. When distressed, the process of reflection-in-action can have a negative bias. Acknowledging this bias and questioning the validity brings the self-awareness of the internal supervisor back into play. For

Advantages of full disclosure of the research protocol	Disadvantages of full disclosure of the research protocol
1. The Relationship between the researcher and the participant	
Facilitates the development of the collaborative relationship with equal partnership in mutually learning from each other. The roles of researcher and participant become inseparable. Through the interactions between the researcher and participant, meaning is created and constructed as an inter-subjective phenomenon (Beck, 1994).	The relationship might become 'pseudotherapeutic, complicating the research process' (Carr, 1994: 718). In the extreme, the role of researcher and participant becoming inseparable where experiences become entangled (Sandelowski, 1996). Wearing two hats, one as nurse and the other as researcher, making the transition from one to the other is fraught with difficulties (Wilde, 1992).
2 Self-disclosure	
Appropriate in modelling the internal supervisor reflecting-in-action. Draws parallels in the multiple roles of supervisor, supervisee and clinician. The use of the self consciously and unconsciously as part of the research process (Swanson, 1986). The use of the self as the main research tool aims to facilitate the disclosure of rich data (Parahoo, 1997, cited in Chambers, 1998: 207).	Need to guard against revealing your own attitudes, opinions and values that might influence the informant's reactions and runs the danger of contaminating the data (Field & Morse, 1985; Beck 1994; Chenitz & Swanson, 1986). The use of bracketing maintains objectivity (Koch, 1998).
3 Engagement	
Engagement through collaboration and inter-personal effectiveness facilitates disclosure in eliciting rich data that proves depth to the inquiry (Wilde, 1992).	Reduces the diversity of data collected. Participants are less likely to be revealing in the absence of engagement in research.
4 Truth	
Truth is an elusive goal, with the experiences lived and perceived by the participants valued as subjective experiences. This is my narrative in researching my own practice. There is no such thing as objective reality (Jasper, 1994). The interpretation of human experience is what is recognised and considered to be true by the participants (Koch, 1994).	Need objective measurement to substantiate the truth in establishing validity and reliably. Viewing truth as illusive makes the research process woolly.
5 The Hawthorn Effect	
Information prior to participating in any type of research involves giving information as part of the ethical considerations. The participant has a pre-reflective experience that involves thinking about the phenomena that is being studied (Jasper, 1994). People will inevitably alter their behaviour in light of new information; however, this is an important part of reflexivity.	The Hawthorn effect needs to be minimised. A simple explanation of the study will maximise the purity of the data.

Figure 4.5   *The advantages and disadvantages of making full disclosure of the research protocol as part of the socialisation process into reflexivity in developing the internal supervisor*

example, the 'cognitive distortion emotional reasoning,' Emma's internal supervisor interpreted emotion as evidence of truth; feeling bad about a situation added up to being, a bad nurse.

In my reflexive case study, cognitive distortions that blocked the internal supervisor were transient: as soon as the unconscious was made conscious the internal supervisor quickly drew from past experiences whilst examining the evidence objectively in reconstructing the situation reflexively. From this experience the concept of multiple levels of reflection was evident, with a relationship between the depth of reflection and the increase of emotional discomfort discovered. For further information on cognitive distortions read Burns (1981).

I am operating under the assumption that the researcher/practitioner needs to become a reflective practitioner through developing their internal supervisor to be effective clinically. This belief is well supported in the literature; Jones (1995) & Johns (1995) promote reflection-in-action that is developed through reflection-on-action as an effective way of developing knowledge. Part of the skill of the clinical supervisor is to draw upon empirical evidence in facilitating the learning process. Examining the work on *Social Learning Theory* (Abrams & Niaura, 1987) three core dimensions to learning are seen in the model of reflective practice. Vicarious capability involves learning through modelling and observing people's behaviour and its consequences; in this sense the supervisor is continually modelling the process of questioning that facilitates reflection. The self-regulatory capability is the capacity to regulate behaviour through internal standards and self-evaluative reactions, an integral part of reflective practice. The third process of learning is the individual's self-reflective capacity to monitor ideas and being an active agent in their own destiny; the clinical supervisor facilitates this in the process of reflection, enabling the practitioner to evaluate and reformulate their thoughts in deciding a course of action.

Atkins & Murphy (1993) discuss the value of experiencing discomfort in clinical supervision, which they perceive as crucial in initiating reflection and self-awareness. Beck et al. (1979) argues that a change in mood or affect shift is a product of automatic thoughts, and that becoming aware of thoughts and emotions (similar to the activation of the internal supervisor) is central to change. Glen et al. (1994) suggest that the activation of critical self-consciousness fosters intellectual growth and behavioural change. The internal supervisor notices vulnerabilities and making the unconscious conscious creates a discomfort that fuels the process of challenging behaviour and hence changing in light of this new information.

Theme 5: Enhancing the internal supervisor: strategies that promote reflexivity

Four key strategies that enhanced reflexivity in promoting the development of the internal supervisor were identified and are summarised in Figure 4.6.

I questioned the common thread that was running through strategies that enhanced the internal supervisor. The process and structure of reflective practice has been influenced by the work of Carper (1978), who described four patterns of 'knowing' in nursing, the empirical, personal, ethical and aesthetic. With the

1   The use of metaphor and story telling in understanding the process of reflexivity.
2   Maintaining a reflective journal and reflexive writing as a medium for reflexivity.
3   Listening to tape recordings of the clinical supervision sessions in developing skills of critical reflection and reflection-in-action through the internal supervisor.
4   Conceptualising the supervisee in recognising vulnerabilities that block the internal supervisor, strategies that develop a positive self-concept to increase trust in reflection-in-action.

Figure 4.6   *A summary of strategies that enhanced reflexivity*

empirical, the internal supervisor draws upon relevant knowledge and evidence for practice. The personal is holistic as the internal supervisor recognises and understands distress. The ethical involves the internal supervisor responding with appropriate skill and action to a situation. The aesthetic way of knowing involves understanding yourself within the context of practice where the internal supervisor questions reflexively faulty assumptions and beliefs that could produce a negative outcome. Enhancing reflexivity is developing the aesthetic way of knowing in nursing, but what about the process of reflexivity itself? Mezirow (1981) described the process of reflection as a multifaceted roundabout in identifying three dimensions that are subdivided into seven dimensions of processing that are on a continuum from developing an awareness of cognition and emotion to greater self-awareness, critical evaluation, analysis and syntheses. The roundabout can be exited and rejoined at any point during the reflective process, just like choosing to take a snapshot or zooming in on a particular scene. But how does knowing this develop the internal supervisor? Rawnsley (cited in Johns and Graham, 1996) proposed that nurses need a conceptual framework of themselves and the supervisor process in which to base their experience that would help make sense of reflection-in-action. Is there a relationship between Mezirow's levels of reflection and a cognitive model based on information processing theory in conceptualising the supervisee? see Figure 4.7.

Both models attempt to highlight differences in how we process information and the relationship between different levels of consciousness. They also strive to help the individual gain insight through critical self-awareness. Mezirow (1981) presents his argument in a very black-and-white way through telling us what we need to know without helping us to understand the reflective process. For example, he states that one must become critically conscious of how our belief systems distort and reflect social, political and moral reality and how that false truth is maintained. By critical reflectivity he is referring to developing a level of awareness of why we attach the meanings and interpretations to reality, roles and relationships, that we do. His statements do not provide the answers but more reflective questions such as 'How do we become aware in developing critical reflection?' For example, in studies about the unpopular patient (Kelly & May 1982; Breeze & Repper, 1998), the patient is categorised as good or bad in terms of their characteristics and not as the nurse practitioner's appraisal of them. How is it possible to all feel the same way about the people that we meet, or to share the same passions in life?

Levels of reflectivity model	Cognitive model
Critical Consciousness • Theoretical reflectivity • Psychic reflectivity • Conceptual reflectivity	Beliefs • Self • Other people • The World • The future
Consciousness • Judgmental reflectivity • Discriminant reflectivity • Affective reflectivity • Reflectivity	Conditional assumptions • Rules • Attitudes
Objects of reflectivity • Perceiving • Thinking • Acting • Habits of perceiving, thinking and acting	Cognitive products • Situation • Thoughts • Emotions • Behaviour

Figure 4.7   *Parallels between Mezirow's model (1981) of reflexivity and Beck et al.'s cognitive model (1979) in conceptualising the supervisee*

Emma held a belief that the doctor always knows best and would notice herself feeling frustrated when she was not listened to. We challenged this belief that enabled her internal supervisor to be more objective in the clinical setting (ethical knowing). In challenging the internal supervisor we needed to build confidence in strengthening the supervisor; metaphor was one way. Froggatt (1998) suggest two approaches to understanding metaphor that she links to an epistemological base. In being consistent with the constuctivist (romantic) epistemology, metaphor in terms of developing reflexivity is seen as central to the conceptualisation of one mental domain to another through a creative force (aesthetics) that provides a way of exploring emotions creatively in reflecting reality.

Metaphor and storytelling is a way of making practice visible through the content of the narrative that aims to place the self within the research process (Koch, 1998). Bringing the internal supervisor into the open within an environment safe to disclosure facilitates growth. Michaels (1995), considering poetry as a further creative source of language, comments that 'the poetry window of ever changing consciousness through which the writers see and readers see the ever changing world' (cited in Holmes & Gregory, 1998: 1192).

Just as reflexive writing expresses the voice of the internal supervisor (Rolfe, 1998), the poet attempts to represent more than the experience.

Consistent throughout reflexive research process and process of writing has been myself as researcher. Theme 6 aims to reflect on myself as researcher during this process.

1   My internal supervisor challenging my lack of faith in qualitative research
    as credible.
2   The internal supervisor helping me adapt in locating myself within the research
    process.
3   Living with uncertainty within the research process.
4   The research process in refining my system as I go along.
5   Analysing the data in deciding what to and what not to include.

Figure 4.8   *Challenges in the research process for the internal*
              supervisor

Theme 6: The internal supervisor in developing the researcher as a
participant self-observer

Central to my reflexive single case study has been reflection on my role as
researcher within the research process, which has taken me on a journey of discovery through exploration of the phenomena of the internal supervisor. I had
several hoops to leap through before reaching this stage and these are summarised
in Figure 4.8.

Rolfe (1998) discusses how the reflexive focus is on both the researcher as participant observer of your own practice (intrapersonal) and as observer of the participant (interpersonal). In qualitative research the researcher is often perceived as
static within the research process in an attempt to adhere to the rules of empirical
research. Jasper (1994) discusses how the researcher preconceptions and experiences might influence the process of the research in a negative way. This is an
integral part of reflexive case study; after all, this is my narrative, both interpersonal and contextual. Making public my preconceptions provides insight in to my
development as researcher. Bracketing my beliefs and prejudices to adopt a
researcher role that involves a selected part of my persona is incongruent with the
aims of my research (Walters, 1995). I brought to the study my multiple roles that
are inseparable from my role as researcher. Modelling my internal supervisor to
Emma in helping her develop and refine her internal supervisor involved a degree
of disclosure on my part and in turn enhanced the research process. Reflecting on
my experience as a developing researcher has been an important part of the
process that enabled my internal supervisor to recognise problems and learn from
them through constantly making modifications to the study and in leading me to
new pastures full of rich information.

Discussion

How does the acquisition insight and self-awareness through the development of
the internal supervisor within the process of reflexivity provide evidence in practice? The content of all the data collected in the reflective case study provided
evidence that the development of the dynamic internal supervisor had a positive

1 Socialisation through education into clinical supervision, reflective practice and reflexive case study.
White et al. (1998) concluded that education and preparation for the role of supervisor is essential in guarding against the danger of supervision been misused as a punitive management tool.

2 Researcher challenging negative beliefs, assumptions and prejudices about qualitative research through (i) operationalising my internal supervisor, (ii) increasing knowledge of relevant philosophies and theories, and (iii) reflecting-on-action in my thesis supervision.
Milton and Ashley (1998) suggest that the supervisor needs to become aware of and explore their negative reactions that are consistent with the existential-phenomenological principle where negative beliefs are dealt with and put aside in becoming reflexive. Playle and Mullarkey (1998) discuss the parallel process in clinical supervision. The supervisor in the role of supervisee who reflects-on-action in their role as supervisor through a cognitive post-mortem in exploring their concerns (Greenwood, 1993: 1185) This process becomes parallel to the supervisor supervising the supervisee, who then repeats this process in the clinical setting, nurse to patient.

3 An assessment of the participant's positive and negative beliefs about clinical supervision, intrapersonal and interpersonal.
Beck (1995), in discussing cognitive therapy assessment, suggests that problems that may inhibit the therapeutic process need to be collaboratively identified and explored before the therapy can proceed. Given that there are parallels in the supervisory relationship and the therapeutic relationship, it is essential to explore this area (Greenwald & Young, 1998; Newman, 1998).

4 Formulation of the participant in recognising strengths and barriers to developing the internal supervisor.
Persons (1989) discusses how a case formulation model conceptualises both the overt difficulties and strengths and the underlying positive and negative psychological mechanisms in identifying barriers to the reflective process.

5 Developing a collaborative therapeutic relationship that built on the positive whilst simultaneously eroding the barriers.
Padesky & Greenberger (1995), in referring to schema theory, stress the importance of simultaneously developing positive self-schema as negative schema are modified. Cust (1995) defined schemas as knowledge structure stored in memory. Given that schema drive cognition, emotion and behaviour, achieving a balance that reinforces achievement whilst modifying the barriers enhances the positive self-concept in developing the internal supervisor.

6 High support, high challenge as a vehicle for change.
Bond & Holland (1998) advocate high support, high challenge in producing changes. Jones (1995) believes the experience of surprise or discomfort in the supervisory relationship initiates the reflective process in activating the internal supervisor.

7 Using affect shifts in identifying the internal supervisor in-action through reflection-on-action to increase awareness of cognitive processes.
Beck et al. (1979) suggests homing in on a person's sudden change in mood to elicit the underlying cognitions. In becoming aware of the thoughts of the internal supervisor, the unconscious becomes conscious.

Continued

8   Sharing the voice of my internal supervisor and personal disclosure, for example, 'What I'm thinking right now is ...'.
    Greenwald and Young in 1998 believe that mutual self-disclosure at a more personal level helps to establish a bond between the supervisor and supervisee.

9   The modelling of clinical supervision skills.
    Cust (1995: 218) said, 'Modelling is a powerful technique for illustrating strategic learning.'

10 Enhancing the development of the internal supervisor through creativity relying on multiple senses, reflexive writing, listening to tapes of sessions, tuning in to bodily sensations and emotions.
    If multiple ways of learning through the senses are adopted, the more likely this awareness is stored in memory (Wells & Matthews, 1994).

11 Analysis of critical incidents through reflection-on-action within the clinical supervision session with a focus on exploring and understanding the reasons why the internal supervisor was ignored. Moving from the specific to the general in identifying themes that inhibit development: for example, the doctor always knows best. Making explicit the reflective spiral.
    Cust (1995) suggested that reflecting-on-action in clinical supervision was increasing meta-cognitive awareness that enhanced the learning process. Through analysis of critical incident, problems can be identified and solved.

Figure 4.9   *A theory of the process in developing the internal supervisor in increasing self-concept and clinical competence*

effect on both clinical care and on increasing a positive self-concept. What was the process? Eleven stages were identified (see Figure 4.9).

Central to the process of developing the self-aware internal supervisor is the articulation of cognition and emotion through vocal expression; this was achieved through the development of a good, collaborative therapeutic alliance. The process began with silence in clinical supervision that had parallels to the clinical environment, and through guided reflection the 'voice' emerged. As clinical supervision sessions progressed the 'voice' of the internal supervisor, amplified as confidence was gained through the empowerment of the supervisee.

Johns and Hardy (1998) draw upon the work of Belenky et al. (1986), referring to the voice as a metaphor. The concept of silence holds negatively-laden assumptions such as impoverished self-expression and subordination. Through reflection the nurse can move along a continuum from silence to assertiveness whilst simultaneously increasing self-esteem. Emma travelled this journey with some discomfort in becoming aware of her internal supervisor, to allowing herself to be guided by it.

Whilst it would be an oversimplification and generalisation to suggest that the development of the internal supervisor improves clinical competence, the findings of this study show the development of my skill as a researcher and clinical supervisor through becoming aware of and operationalising my internal supervisor. Through tracking my internal supervisor and the exploration of evidence enabled me to overcome potential difficulties. Emma believed that her clinical practice had been transformed through the development of her internal supervisor through reflection-on-action in clinical supervision. She moved from a position as sceptic to advocator of clinical supervision, having both personally and professionally reaped its benefits. She is now on the road to becoming a clinical supervisor herself, with a hope of helping her colleagues experience some of her learnings.

The internal supervisor is dynamic and ongoing in its clinical development, constantly analysing and evaluating reactions to new situations and bringing new experiences and information to old familiar situations. The end is an elusive goal as the process of reflexivity is circular (Rolfe, 1998).

References

Abrams, D.B. & Niaura, R.S. (1987) *Social Learning Theory.* New York: Guilford Press.

Allen, R.E. (1993) *The Concise Oxford Dictionary of Current English.* 8th edn. Oxford: Oxford University Press.

Atkins, S. & Murphy, K. (1993) 'Reflection: a review of the literature'. *Journal of Advanced Nursing,* **18** (11), 88–1192.

Beck, A.T., Freeman, A. & Associates (1990) *Cognitive Therapy of Personality Disorders.* Guilford Press: New York.

Beck, A., Rush, J.A., Shaw, B.F. & Emery, G. (1979) *Cognitive Therapy of Depression.* Guilford Press: New York.

Beck, C.T. (1994) 'Phenomenology: its use in nursing research'. *International Journal of Nursing Studies,* **31** (6), 499–510.

Beck, J.S. (1995) *Cognitive Therapy Basics and Beyond.* Guilford Press: New York.

Belenky, M.F., Clinchy, B.M., Goldberger, N.R. & Tarule, J.M. (1986) *Women's Ways of Knowing.* New York: Basic Books.

Bond, M. & Holland, S. (1998) *Skills of Clinical Supervision for Nurses.* Milton Keynes: Open University Press.

Breeze, J.A. & Repper, J. (1998) 'Struggling for control: the care experiences of "difficult" patients in mental health services'. *Journal of Advanced Nursing,* **28** (6), 1301–1311.

Burns, D.D. (1981) *Feeling Good: The New Mood Therapy.* Penguin Books: New York.

Butterworth, T. (1994) 'Preparing to take on clinical supervision'. *Nursing Standard,* **8** (52), 32–4.

Carper, B. (1978) 'Fundamental patterns of knowing in nursing'. *Advances in Nursing Science,* **1** (1), 13–23.

Carr, L.T. (1994) 'The strengths and weaknesses of qualitative and quantitative research: what method for nursing'. *Journal of Advanced Nursing,* **20**: 4, 716–21.

Casement, P. (1985) *On Learning From the Patient.* New York: Guilford Press.

Chambers, M. (1995) 'Supportive clinical supervision a crucible for personal and professional change'. *Journal of Psychiatric and Mental Health Nursing,* **2**: 4, 311–16.

Chambers, M. (1998) 'Interpersonal mental health nursing: research issues and challenges'. *Journal of Psychiatric and Mental Health Nursing,* **5**: 3, 203–211.

Chenitz, W.C. & Swanson, J.M. (1986) (eds) *From Practice to Grounded Theory: Qualitative Research in Nursing.* California: Addison Wesley.

Clark, D.A. (1997) 'Is cognitive therapy ill founded? A commentary on Lyddon and Weill'. *Journal of Cognitive Psychotherapy,* **11** (2), 91–7.

Cust, J. (1995) 'Recent cognitive perspectives on learning: implications for nurse education'. *Nurse Education Today*, **15**: 4, 280–90.

Cutcliffe, J.R. & Proctor, B. (1998a) 'An alternative training approach to clinical supervision: 2'. *British Journal of Nursing*, **7** (6), 344–50.

Cutcliffe, J.R. & Proctor, B. (1998b) 'An alternative training approach to clinical supervision: 1'. *British Journal of Nursing*, **7** (5), 281–5.

Department of health (1993) *A Vision for the Future: the nursing, midwifery and health visiting contribution to health and health care.* London: HMSO.

Devine, A. (1995) 'Introducing clinical supervision: a guide'. *Nursing Standard*, **28** (40), 32–3.

Epstein, S. (1998) *Constructive thinking: the key to emotional intelligence.* Praeger Publishing: Connecticut.

Farrington, A. (1998) 'Clinical supervision: issues for mental health nursing'. *Mental Health Nursing*, **18** (1), 19–21.

Field, P.A. and Morse, J.M. (1985) *Nursing Research.* London: Chapman and Hall.

Fowler, J. (1995) 'Nurses perceptions of the elements of good supervision'. *Nursing Times*, **91** (22), 33–7.

Freshwater, D. (1998) 'Transformatory Learning in Nurse Education'. Unpublished PhD Thesis. University of Nottingham.

Friedman, S. & Marr, J. (1995) 'A supervisory model of professional competence: a joint service education initiative'. *Nurse Education Today*, **15**: 4 239–44.

Froggatt, K. (1998) 'The place of metaphor and language in exploring nurses' emotional work'. *Journal of Advanced Nursing*, **28** (2), 332–8.

Gergen, K.J. and Gergen, M.M. (1991) 'From theory to reflexivity in research pratice', in Steiner, F. (ed.) *Method and Reflexivity: knowing as systemic social construction.* London: Sage, pp. 76–95.

Glen, S., Clark, A. & Nicol, M. (1994) 'Reflecting on reflection: a personal encounter'. *Nurse Education Today*, **15**: 2, 61–8.

Greenberger, D. (1992) 'The suicidal patient'. in Freeman, A. & Dattilio, F.M. (eds) *Comprehensive Casebook of Cognitive Therapy.* New York: Plenum Press: Ch. 13.

Greenwald, M. & Young, J. (1998) 'Schema-focussed therapy: an integrated approach to psychotherapy supervision'. *Journal of Cognitive Psychotherapy*, **12** (2), 109–126.

Greenwood, J. (1993) 'Reflective practice: a critique of the work of Argris and Schon'. *Journal of Advanced Nursing*, **18**: 1, 1183–7.

Hawkins, P. & Shohet, R. (1989) *Supervision in the Helping Profession*, Milton Keynes: Open University Press.

Heath, H. (1998) 'Paradigm dialogues and dogma: finding a place for research, nursing models and reflective practice'. *Journal of Advanced Nursing*, **28** (2), 288–94.

Hilliard, R.B., Strupp, H.H. & Henry, W.P. (2000) 'An interpersonal model of psychotherapy linking patient and therapist developmental history, therapeutic process and types of outcome'. *Journal of Consulting and Clinical Psychology*, **68** (1), 125–33.

Holmes, V. & Gregory, D. (1998) 'Writing poetry: a way of knowing nursing'. *Journal of Advanced Nursing*, **28** (6), 1191–4.

Jasper, M.A. (1994) 'Issues in phenomenology for researchers of nursing'. *Journal of Advanced Nursing*, **19**: 2, 309–314.

Johns, C. (1993) 'Professional supervision'. *Journal of Nursing Management*, **1**: 1, 9–18.

Johns, C. (1995) 'The value of reflective practice for nursing'. *Journal of Clinical Nursing*, **4**: 1, 23–30.

Johns, C. & Freshwater, D. (1998) *Transforming Nursing Through Reflective Practice.* Oxford: Blackwell Science.

Johns, C. & Graham, J. (1996) 'Using a reflective model of nursing and guided reflection'. *Nursing Standard*, **11** (2), 34–8.

Johns, C. & Hardy, H. (1998) 'Voice as a metaphor for transformation through reflective practice', in Johns, C. & Freshwater, D. *Transforming Nursing Through Reflective Practice.* Oxford: Blackwell Science. Ch. 5.

Jones, P.R. (1995) 'Hindsight bias in reflective practice: an empirical investigation'. *Journal of Advanced Nursing*, **21**: 4, 783–8.

Kelly, M.P. & May D. (1982) 'Good and bad patients: a review of the literature and theoretical critique'. *Journal of Advanced Nursing*, **7**: 2, 147–56.

King, E. (1996) 'The use of the self in qualitative research' in Richardson, T.J.E. (ed.) *Handbook of Qualitative Research Methods for Psychology and the Social Sciences.* Leicester: British Psychological Society Books. Ch. 13.

Koch, T. (1994) 'Establishing rigor in qualitative research: the decision trail'. *Journal of Advanced Nursing*, **19**: 5, 976–86.

Koch, T. (1998) 'Story telling: is it really research?' *Journal of Advanced Nursing*, **28** (6), 1182–90.

Liese, B.S. & Alford, B.A. (1998) 'Recent advances in cognitive therapy supervision'. *Journal of Cognitive Psychotherapy*, **12** (2), 91–4.

Lyddon, W.J. & Weill, R. (1997) 'Cognitive psychotherapy and postmodernism: emerging themes and challenges'. *Journal of Cognitive Psychotherapy*, **11** (2), 75–90.

Martin, D.J., Garske, J.P. & Davis, K.M. (2000) 'Relation of the therapeutic alliance and other variables: A meta-analytic review'. *Journal of Consulting and Clinical Psychology*, **68** (3), 438–50.

Mezirow, J. (1981) 'A critical theory of adult learning and education'. *Adult Education,* **32** (1), 3–24.

Milton, M. & Ashley, S. (1998) 'Personal accounts of supervision: phenomenological reflections on "effectiveness"'. *Counselling*, **9**: 4, 311–14.

Munroe, H. (1988) 'Modes of operation in clinical supervision: how clinical supervisors perceive themselves'. *British Journal of Occupational Therapy*, **51** (10), 338–42.

Newman, C.F. (1998) 'Therapeutic and supervisory relationships in cognitive and behavioural psychotherapies: similarities and differences'. *Journal of Cognitive Psychotherapy*, **12** (2), 95–108.

Northcott, N. (1996) 'Supervise to grow': *Nursing Management.* pp. **2** (10), 19–21.

Padesky, C.A. & Greenberger, D. (1995) *A Clinicians Guide to Mind Over Mood.* New York: Guilford Press.

Paolo, S.B. (1998) 'Receiving supervision in cognitive therapy: A personal account'. *Journal of Cognitive Psychotherapy*, **12** (2), 153–62.

Persons, J.B. (1989) *Cognitive Therapy in Practice: A case formulation approach*: New York: Norton.

Playle, J.F. & Mullarkey, K. (1998) 'Parallel processes in clinical supervision: enhancing learning and providing support'. *Nurse Education Today*, **18**: 6, 558–66.

Potter, J. (1996) 'Discourse analyses and constructionist approaches: theoretical background' in Richardson, J.T.E. (ed.) *Handbook of Qualitative Research Methods for Psychology and the Social Sciences.* Leicester: British Psychological Society Books. Ch. 10.

Rogers, C. (1951) *Client-centred Therapy.* Boston: Houghton Mifflin.

Rolfe, G. (1997) 'Writing ourselves: creating knowledge in a postmodern world'. *Nurse Education Today*, **17** (6), 442–8.

Rolfe, G. (1998) *Expanding Nursing Knowledge: Understanding and Researching Your Own Practice.* Oxford: Butterworth Heinemann.

Safran. J.D. & Muran, C.J. (2000) *Negotiating the Therapeutic Alliance: A Relational Treatment Guide.* New York: Guilford Press.

Sandelowski, M. (1986) 'The problem of rigor in qualitative research'. *Advances in Nursing Science*, **8** (3), 27–37.

Schön, D.A (1983) *The Reflective Practitioner.* London: Basic Books.

Stokoe, B. & McClarey, M. (1995) 'Safety measures'. *Nursing Times*, 28 (26), 30–31.

Swanson, J.M. (1986) 'The formal qualitative interview for grounded theory' in Chenitz, W.C. & Swanson, J.M. (eds) *From Practice to Grounded Theory.* Menlow Park California: Addison Wesley.

Titchen, A. & Binnie, A. (1995) 'The art of clinical supervision'. *Journal of Clinical Nursing,* **4** (4), 327–34.

Walters, A.J. (1995) 'The phenomenological movement: implications for nursing research'. *Journal of Advanced Nursing,* **22**: 4, 791–9.

Wells, A. & Matthew, G. (1994) *Attention and Emotion: A Clinical Perspective.* Hove: Lawrence Erlbaum.

White, E., Butterworth, T., Bishop, V., Jeacock, J. & Clements, A. (1998) 'Clinical supervision: insider reports of a private world'. *Journal of Advanced Nursing,* **28** (1), 185–92.

Wilde, V. (1992) 'Controversial hypotheses on the relationship between researcher and informant in qualitative research'. *Journal of Advanced Nursing,* **17**: 2, 234–42.

Zuroff, D.C., Scotsky, S.M., Martin, J.D., Sanislow III, C.A., Blatt, S.J., Krupnick, J.L. & Simmens, S. (2000) 'Relation of the therapeutic alliance and perfectionism to outcome in brief outpatient treatment of depression'. *Journal of Consulting and Clinical Psychology,* **68** (1), 114–24.

PART II

THE EDUCATIONALIST'S PERSPECTIVE

Dawn Freshwater

Recent developments in general education, nursing practice and nursing education, not least the shift into higher education, have influenced the expansion of the nursing curricula significantly. Whilst there is no space here to discuss this in any detail, I will dwell for a moment on one particular movement, which is of direct relevance to the chapters in this Part, that of student-centred learning. Educationalists, nurses and the like have explored student-centred learning and its practical implications *ad infinitum* (see, for example, Askew & Carnell, 1998; Brandes & Ginnis, 1986; Field & Fitzgerald, 1998; Freshwater, 2002; Freshwater, 1998; Knowles, 1970; Rogers, 1983). However, one particular statement that is pertinent to this discussion is written by McMahon, who simply states that 'The preparation of nurses to act therapeutically should be the focus of pre-registration training' (1998: 15). Does student-centred learning, in its approach to education, prepare and enable nursing students to practice therapeutic nursing?

Student-centred learning is based upon the client-centred approach to psychotherapy founded by Carl Rogers (1961). Client-centred care as a term is itself now widely recognised in the domain of nursing and healthcare, particularly of late where we are party to an increasing drive towards consumer involvement in decision making at all levels. The role of the teacher in student-centred learning is that of facilitator of learning experiences; this role is seen as crucial to the development of self-efficacy. As Bandura (1995) comments, students do not just need to know what it is that will make them successful, they need to feel the experience of success. From this perspective self-efficacy, as discussed in Chapter 1, is closely linked to self-esteem and self-regard.

Askew and Carnell contend that the goal of the student-centred model of education is to 'enable young people to fit into society rather than to challenge social injustice' (1998: 89). Building on the client-centred framework proposed by Rogers (1961), they argue that a 'liberatory' approach to education goes someway to redeeming this crucial omission (Friere, 1972). Other writers, having developed this notion in nursing, argue for a transformative and emancipatory model of education. In Chapter 5, Jacqueline Randle provides an insight into the concept of transformative learning (Askew & Carnell, 1998; Freshwater, 2002; Freshwater, 1998), signposting the pitfalls in assisting the pre-registration student nurse to maintain and develop their self-esteem.

Transformative learning not only enables students to learn, and to learn how to learn, but also facilitates the process of transformation in that learning. This process involves a risk for both the student and the facilitator as they undertake to reveal more of who they are, realising the boundaries of their therapeutic potential. Jacqueline refers to this process of revelation as discovering the authentic self. But, if there is an authentic self, how safe is it for that self to be visible? And does nurse education create an environment within which students can feel safe to be authentic? Jacqueline's chapter points to some of the difficulties that student nurses (and indeed other practitioners) face when negotiating their way through the maze of everyday practice. Using examples of students being asked to perform observations on patients that were already dead, Jacqueline refers to Meissner's (1986) notion of 'insidious cannibalism', which has similarities with horizontal violence, that it would seem is rife in nursing (Freshwater, 2000; Leap, 1997; McCall, 1996). Where nurses feel oppressed and ridiculed they are not going to engage their authentic self, rather they will keep themselves protected from public view for fear of shame, preferring to experience a sense of personal meaninglessness. As nurse educators, then, we too have a therapeutic role and it is this that is the pivotal point for Part II of this book. It will become clear that it is imperative that we act as role models of therapeutic practice to our students. As such educationalists, who aim to utilise themselves as a therapeutic tool, are also required to engage in critical reflection in and on their practice.

Higgs and Titchen (2001) argue for the expression of the authentic self in education, stating that 'If we can express our authentic selves, then we can access our creativity and through that realise our life dreams' (2001: 270). Developing this theme, they illustrate how the creative arts and humanities might be used in helping the authentic self to find expression. Field and Fitzgerald (1998) also posit that curriculum writers should strive to discover and develop techniques which are most conducive to learning the skills of communication and understanding the human condition. Art, they recommend, is one such medium for 'both understanding the human condition and communicating with each other at an emotional level'; further, 'it has a great deal to offer nursing students and other caring professions in terms of establishing caring relationships with therapeutic intent and effect' (Field & Fitzgerald, 1998: 105).

Chapter 6 exemplifies the effective use of the creative arts in establishing caring values and beliefs for the enhancement of the therapeutic alliance. Marilyn Parker's illustration of therapeutic education highlights opportunities for expression of aesthetic nursing through facilitation of clay workshops in which nurses are challenged to revisit the core values of their caring practice. As is the case with many art forms, clay sculptures can be used to express the appearance of things, the reality of things, as a way of exploring the unknown or of embodying ideals. Marilyn uses her experience as a potter to enable the participants to use clay as an embodiment of their nursing values.

According to Bruderle and Valiga (1994), poetry, one of the earliest art forms, is thought to have magical powers in many cultures. It is deemed to be a way of capturing the nature of being, allowing both the reader and the author to delve into human experiences. With the absence of rights and wrongs, it is an imaginative approach to education and caring, enabling the expression of feelings and thoughts and emotions. Poems can be free-flowing or more structured, as in the case of the Haiku. This 700-year-old art form consisting of 17 syllables expressed in three lines (5, 7 and 5 syllables respectively), are simple to compose and can be used to evaluate or summarise particular experiences.

Lynne Wagner describes the process of using poetry and art within reflective practice in order to develop the caring self. These chapters raise a number of challenges for nurse educators, firstly related to assignments. That assignments need to be linked to reflection on self and development of self as a professional is not contended here, however, as an educator who has been striving to implement a narrative-based curriculum, one of my deepest frustrations is not the assignments themselves but the appropriate assessment of the same. I know that this is an issue for many educationalists wishing to remain true to the transformative approach to learning, and one that is only just beginning to be addressed. A further problem relates to group size. Lynne speaks of the opportunities for small group process work; this is difficult given the current climate of nurse education, where Diploma groups are often more than 100 and teaching is often shared with key lectures across several disciplines. So the challenge for educationalists and practitioners is to be creative in finding ways of valuing the added dimension that art, the poem, the sculpture can offer to therapeutic nursing and to view learning as a therapeutic tool in itself.

References

Askew, S. & Carnell, E. (1998) *Transformatory Learning: individual and global change*. London: Cassell.

Bandura, A. (1995) 'Exercise of personal and collective efficacy in changing societies' in Bandura, A. (ed.) *Self-efficacy in Changing Societies*. Cambridge: Cambridge University Press.

Brandes, P.L. & Ginnis, P. (1986) *A Guide to Student-centred Learning*. Oxford: Basil Blackwell.

Bruderle, E.R. & Valiga, T.M. (1994) 'Integrating Arts and Humanities into Nurse Education' in Chinn, P.L. and Watson, J. (eds) *Art and Aesthetics in Nursing*. New York: National League for Nursing. Ch. 6.

Field, J. & Fitzgerald, M. (1998) 'Therapeutic Nursing: emerging imperatives for nursing curricula' in McMahon, R. & Pearson, A. (eds) *Nursing as Therapy*. Cheltenham: Stanley Thornes.

Freshwater, D. (2002) 'Transformatory Learning: A postmodern analysis'. *Curriculum Inquiry*. Spring 2002.

Freshwater, D. (2000) 'Cross currents: against cultural narration'. *Journal of Advanced Nursing*, **32** (2), 481–4.

Freshwater, D. (1998) 'Transformatory learning in nurse education'. Unpublished PhD Thesis. University of Nottingham.

Friere, P. (1972) *Pedagogy of the Oppressed.* Harmondsworth: Penguin.

Higgs, J. & Titchen, A. (2001) 'Professional Practice: walking alone with others' in Higgs, J. & Titchen, A. (eds) *Professional Practice in Health, Education and the Creative Arts.* Oxford: Blackwell Science. Ch. 21.

Knowles, M.S. (1970) *The Adult Learner, a neglected species.* 4th edn. Houston: Gulf.

Leap, N. (1997) 'Making sense of "horizontal violence" in midwifery'. *British Journal of Nursing,* **5**: 6, 689.

McCall, E. (1996) 'Horizontal violence in nursing: the continuing silence'. *The Lamp.* April 29–31.

McMahon, R. (1998) 'Therapeutic Nursing, theory, issues and practice' in McMahon, R. & Pearson, A. (eds) *Nursing as Therapy.* Cheltenham: Stanley Thornes.

Meissner, J. (1986) 'Nurses: are we eating our young?' *Nursing,* **16** (3), 51–3.

Rogers, C.R. (1983) *Freedom to Learn in the 80's.* Ohio: Charles Merrill.

Rogers, C.R. (1961) *On Becoming a Person.* Boston: Houghton.

5 Transformative Learning: Enabling Therapeutic Nursing

Jacqueline Randle

Barber argues: 'Show me how well you share of yourself, are able to communicate this to others, and I'll know how good or bad your nursing care is' (1993: 345). Bloom also states: 'We are told the healthy inner-directed person will really care for others'; unfortunately Bloom continues 'To which I can only respond: If you believe that you believe anything' (1987: 178).

These conflicting views ground the rationale for this chapter. Theorists suggest that nurses with a healthy sense of self derived from their self-esteem, are able to share some of themselves with patients and colleagues and subsequently affect patient care in a positive direction (Arthur & Thorne, 1998; Freshwater, 1998; Carson et al., 1997; Olsen, 1995; Reeve, 2000; and Randle, 2001). They also note that nurses who haven't a healthy sense of self affect the quality of care in a negative direction. A positive sense of self means that people feel good about themselves, and as people become more positive about themselves, they become more positive about others (Andersson, 1993). In healthcare, this generally results in facilitation of sound, interpersonal relationships not only with patients, but also with carers and colleagues.

Unfortunately, although students and nurses may commence nursing with a healthy sense of self, working environments often hamper the ability to use self therapeutically (Freshwater, 2000; Reeve, 2000; Randle, 2001). It may be, as Bloom's comment suggests, that in nursing, students and nurses may have to adopt a false self in order to cope with the demands of their role. The challenge to educators is to transform practice whereby a situation exists that students and nurses may wish to be authentic and share something of themselves. However, the context they find themselves in often demands acculturation to a different way of working, which can be detrimental to patients, themselves and nursing generally. This chapter examines the pressures facing students and nurses in their everyday practice and provides examples of the conflicts between the desire to be authentic and therapeutic with the realities of nursing work. These narratives arose from interviewing two cohorts of students who were undertaking a three-year diploma in nursing course in a higher education establishment in the UK. Students were interviewed at the beginning and end of their course and openly shared their stories with me, the practitioner/researcher. These were rich sources of experience, describing how students felt about their journeys to becoming a nurse and included insights into how both nurses and students use their self in their everyday nursing work.

The healthy self

In order to provide effective, humanistic nursing care, students and nurses should have a healthy sense of self. Characteristics of a healthy sense of self include the use of the authentic-self, empathy, the delivery of individualised, holistic care and continuing in the face of adversity. Reynolds and Scott (2000) emphasise the importance of relationship development and therapeutic communication in nursing practice. Ulrich (1996) states that to care for others a person firstly has to care for themselves; this requires an understanding of the self as well as the person being cared for. Similarly, to be able to value patients and clients, students and nurses have to be able to value themselves first and part of this process is being self-aware (Cook, 1999). This implies that students and nurses should have a sound personal identity. An important aspect of identity is not only defining one-self in a relationship, but also defining how to go about caring for the other in the relationship. Both personal and professional identities are important components of a healthy sense of self and this is enhanced when nurses develop a deep valuing commitment to themselves (Bunkers, 1992). A positive self-image as a reflection of professional self is a prerequisite for students and nurses to be able to have a strong and therapeutic relationship with the patient. The professional self is developed through the process of becoming a nurse. Previous work (Freshwater, 1998; Arthur, 1992) has suggested that there is a continuing problem with nurses' self-esteem and that the professional self is low. It would appear that nurses are experiencing an inability to exert control over their professional environment, and subsequently, feelings of social devaluation and feelings of loss of autonomy are common amongst them. This has been documented in the nursing literature (Bullivent, 1998) and, in my personal experience, the cry of 'morale has never been so low' is common. The impact this context has on patient care and the use of therapeutic self is well-documented elsewhere (Briant & Freshwater, 1998; Higgs & Titchen, 2001; McMahon & Pearson, 1998). A common conflict facing nurses is between the need for them to have the attributes of a healthy self on the one hand, but on the other, being left to acquire these themselves.

The context of where students begin to identify with and develop their professional self is central to any developments in the use of self as a therapeutic tool. Findings from interviews with students showed that it was evident that the primary influence on the development of the professional self was nurses in the clinical area (Reeve, 2000). Central to any developments in the professional self is the notion that the sense of self is largely, if not entirely constructed through interaction with and feedback from significant others (Terry et al., 1999). Other theorists also argue that the self has its genesis within the social group (Hogg & Abrams, 1990; Meeres & Grant, 1999). The desire for consistency is a central motivator of human conduct (Cialdini et al., 1999). Richness in feedback from the wider social context makes it virtually impossible not to self-compare. Social comparison, then, plays a central role in maintaining the professional self. In order to enhance the self in the eyes of other nurses, it is likely that students and nurses will conform to the roles and standards expected of them.

Part of this conformity is the assimilation of professional norms, commonly referred to as professional socialisation. Mozingo et al. (1995) have referred to this process as students having to 'pass the tribal test'. This may not be as extreme as scenarios described in Alavi and Cattoni's (1995) paper, where students described being asked to take observations on patients who the rest of the staff knew were already dead. However, in its most severe form the socialisation process can be akin to brainwashing and Meissner (1986) alleges that nursing faculties are guilty of 'insidious cannibalism' due to socialisation processes that change students' personalities. Du Toit's (1995) study of first and third year Australian nursing students in two universities, found that the majority of students conformed so much that their nursing identity subsumed how they felt about themselves as being female, or married and so on. Unfortunately contextual influences, that is, nursing culture, can be so great that students seemingly feel that their professional self requires validation by nurses to give them a reality. In order to enhance the professional self in the eyes of others, it is likely that students and nurses will conform to the roles and standards expected of them. This means that students and nurses adopt norms, values and rules that are characterised by working as a member of the collective nursing group.

Sometimes, then, the process of becoming a nurse can have a detrimental effect on the student. Cultural factors conspire to force many students and nurses to compromise their authentic 'selves', an adaptation that takes its toll in other arenas in their lives. This is a consequence of practitioners not always being able to work in ways that they wish. This impacts on the practitioner's sense of self. If conflict exists between the type of care students and nurses wish to provide and that they actually perform, negative self-evaluative beliefs may result (Reeve, 2000). This was the case for the students I interviewed. Although the majority of students that participated in the study started their course with normal self-esteem, by the end of the course their self-esteem had decreased in such a way that 95 per cent of them had below-normal self-esteem. The socialisation process affected how they felt about themselves, so that the majority felt anxious, depressed and were unable to act towards patients and colleagues in a therapeutic manner. For the students involved in the study it was a hard price to pay in order to gain professional status, as their self was fragmented and their personal resources depleted.

The status of being a student is in itself confusing, as multiple boundaries have to be crossed in a short pace of time. In extreme circumstances students can go through a divestiture process in which the organisation attempts to strip individuals of their identity in order for them to comply with the needs of the organisation. The transitory situation of becoming a nurse, disorientation, lack of personal identity and an inadequate role identity ensure that students are more susceptible to divestiture. Divestiture processes generally go on in an unrecognisable manner to those who are already part of the socialisation process, and most people are unconscious of the fact that they may be contributing to this process. It appears, then, that the socialisation process may affect the personal and professional self, in that it is likely that students lose something of themselves in order to identify with being a nurse. Of course, students can be equally susceptible to the investiture process, where socialisation helps to confirm the identity of the student in order to raise self-esteem and thus the use of therapeutic self.

The valuing of the student as an individual gains more significance when reviewing literature that suggests that those students who are able to retain some personal identity through their relationships outside work have higher self-esteem (Mozingo et al., 1995). Carson et al.'s (1997) study surveyed 245 community mental health nurses and 323 ward-based mental health nurses in a health authority in England. A comprehensive range of questionnaires assessing levels of general health, burnout, self-esteem and job satisfaction and coping skills alongside demographic variables were utilised. Results supported prior work in that self-esteem was significantly higher in staff who were happy in their life, were fit, had job security, had supportive relationships with line managers and who had children.

When students are befriended and treated as individuals, they generally retain a healthy degree of authentic self and will be more likely to be therapeutic in their work. Spouse's (1996) longitudinal study following eight students over a four-year period showed that befriending was the key to all other learning activities. If the students were not befriended they became invisible, ignored and idle and were left to their own devices. The importance of the mentor making the first step in helping the student feel welcomed and valued is unequivocal. Clinical learning in preparation to become a nurse has long been acknowledged to be significant (White, 1996). Unfortunately, student support and maintenance of students' personal identities has often been a haphazard affair due to student's intense workload commitment and the lack of qualified staff available to support them (Spouse, 1996). Consequently, students are often left to themselves in their formal search for a professional self. Rogers (1951) believes that human beings have a need for positive self-regard, which is universally learned through experiences with parents. If nurses treat students with unconditional regard, they develop a healthy sense of self. Conversely, if students are treated with conditional regard, they suffer with a low sense of self.

Unfortunately, mentors may be in a powerless position themselves and thus be thwarted in their therapeutic sense of self. Students in my study expressed that a common occurrence in their experiences was the power nurses had over them. For instance, Jenny, who was nearing the end of her course, reported:

> I think I've learnt when to speak and when not to, when to ask questions and also the sort of questions you do ask. I think it's alright, it's like speaking when you're spoken to.

Repeated negative actions such as this had an impact on the sense of self and occurred because of being in the social position of student in the nursing hierarchy. Due to the way students felt about themselves after such negative experiences, they typically conformed to the norms and values that existed, as they became powerless to challenge them. Students found common experiences of learning in the clinical areas were as a consequence of custodial, authoritarian ways of nursing practice.

An extract from an interview with Victoria exemplifies this:

> You were a waste of time as far as the staff were concerned. The patients like you and they respect the fact you're there, just talking. They'd say, 'Oh the nurses haven't got

time to talk to us.' I know nurses are busy but surely they've got time to say 'Hello, how are you?' Some nurses did, the NA's (nursing auxiliaries) more than the trained staff. I had a few problems getting on with staff. I didn't think they could be all that bad, but then I realised what they were like. That's what worries me about going up to X; it's the staff that have the problems, not the patients. I'm the kind of person who'd like to say something but I don't think you can. It depends what ward you're on. I don't get upset, I just get annoyed and I can't ignore it. I can't go to bed annoyed 'cos I can't sleep and then I wake up even more annoyed. So I think I'd have to go and speak to someone, someone above them without sounding too much as if I'm telling tales. There's something that has to be done to get it sorted out to see why they're being this way to me.

The lack of general support by nursing staff in clinical areas affected Victoria's self-esteem. Victoria was hurt and upset by her experiences of training that caused her interrupted sleep and emotional turmoil. She wanted help from someone in authority to stop what was happening to her, but yet was 'scared to go to teacher telling tales' due to the repercussions she perceived she would face.

This negative experience was not unique to Victoria; Colette states:

It's like Jane on *X* ward, the Sister said really loudly, 'Does this student have a name then?' And that was that for the day. So a few of us have met the dreaded Sister. So they tell you to be good and if you don't want to do it, then don't do it. But we're afraid it will go against us and that's one of my worries, if I say I don't want to do something, how is that going to affect my reference? Are we there to be slaves? You tend to fall in and do whatever.

A typical reaction to such experiences was passivity and conformity.

To maintain a sense of nurse identity, students seemed to work hard at fitting in and maintaining the *status quo* in order to make other nurses more positively responsive to them. They then felt more positive about themselves as would-be nurses.

When students were able to reflect on their training, there was a greater awareness that nurses exercised power over students. The most extreme comment was made by Gill:

I wouldn't do it over again, no, not this. If I knew what it was going to be, I don't know, but I definitely wouldn't do this again. I never thought nurses could be so bitchy. I'm a grown woman and they've made my life hell, really. My daughter's at school and she's had less bullying than me. They're just bullies, to other nurses and to the patients as well. They ought to be sacked.

Susan, reflecting on her experiences, told me:

Not so much here, but when I was on ward X and I think, ward X, you get to that stage and you go on to the ward and the staff nurses say you can do this and you can do that and like we turn round and say we can't because we've never done it before. They make you feel really stupid, but what can you do? If you haven't done it then you haven't done it.

Emily continues this theme:

Generally, I thought they were OK ... they've been OK. I had a problem with X ward, but it never got resolved. I had a problem with regards to working every single weekend for the three months I was down there, apart from one and the fact I got treated ... mainly by the Sister, but some of the staff nurses as well, as if I was something that had crawled out of underneath a stone. And you know like, all the placements you talk about other things apart from work but at X they never really spoke to you except, 'Can you go and do this?' and 'Do that' and 'Have you done this?', 'Have you done that?' It really was hard down there. It never really got resolved and I know the students before me got problems, and I know the student down there now and she's got problems so I think something should be done there ... Yes, well, you got used to working weekends and a social life went out of the window but you accepted it, but apart from the way they spoke to you and the way they made you feel, that was the worst bit. I think it was just because I was a student.

A different student, Tara, reflects a similar theme in that:

Some of the staff nurses there do have problems, I think it is just one of them wards. It's not very good to go to and as a student with regards to your learning down there, you take pot luck really. I mean, fair enough, they are short staffed, but you're still a student at the end of the day. You're not there to make up for their lack of staff, you're there to learn. But they didn't seem to get that across. If I'd had another placement as bad as X I think I would have packed my bags. You know I was just there as an auxiliary, which is fair enough, you don't mind doing that but at the end of the day, you have still got to balance your learning with other things.

On one of Suzy's wards, which was an adult branch placement, she described how on practice they had nursing and medical personnel from the Navy:

They treated me like a naval personnel because I was down there and obviously I'm not, so I don't think that was so good really and they spoke to me like I was, you know, they are very stern aren't they? The Sisters, they are really quite frightening at times. I don't know if this was good for me or not really. If I was in the Navy fair enough but because I'm not it doesn't apply to me does it?

Another student, Kerry, reflected on her three years of training for mental health registration and told me:

I've been told to act less like a student and more like a qualified nurse, because if I was one tomorrow, I wouldn't be able to change overnight. I think it's my confidence, it depends who you work with and I suppose I'm quite sensitive to the way other people act towards me. I think it's my problem not theirs, but sometimes when I'm on an off-day it makes my confidence go down. I don't like bugging people all the time, but then again I didn't like, just go on and get on with things in case I'm doing something I've already done or if they're not happy with me doing something. It's hard to get in with them and I always feel I'm apologising for nothing really ... I think ... I don't know.

Nurses devaluing students because of their lack of practical experience or apparent lack of knowledge was a theme reiterated by others. Sharon reflects on her first placement in a hospital:

I think the first placement up here, they were, they expected more of you. I had sort of occasions when people would turn around and say, 'Well, don't you know this' and I would think well no, I don't, and they would be like off and I would think well you never shown me or I didn't know.

These reflections portray that many students experienced negative situations, which affected their self-esteem. For some students, the fact that they had not taken any action to protect themselves or those who were in a more vulnerable position resulted in negative emotional states such as anger, anxiety and stress. One student expressed the belief that she 'didn't like herself much' and this was a theme that was initially expressed by students. With the exception of anecdotal literature in the nursing press, this oppressive, bullying type of nursing had not been documented prior to the findings of this study. The students, who were on the receiving end of such tactics, legitimately found these very distressing. However, instead of challenging such practices, they chose to try to continue with their placement, knowing that it would soon be over. This strategy seemed to be the only one that could ensure that they would continue with the course, which is what the majority were determined to do. Interestingly, they then went on to participate in similar activities, which encouraged the patient to be placed in vulnerable positions.

The social structure in which nursing operates ensures that students are placed in a precarious position, as they know the actions of the nurses are sometimes wrong, yet at the same time feel powerless to act due to their position in the hierarchy. This is where learning from a role model is not always beneficial, as nurses' attitudes towards colleagues are often followed from expediency. It would be easy to criticise students in these situations, yet the context in which learning occurs may define their relative powerlessness. Students who offered these accounts during interviews were relatively new in their student-nurse trajectory and were under great pressure to comply with the wishes of the nursing staff. They were also aware that staff had to complete a practice assessment document that would affect their progression on the course. Similarly, trained nurses may act in such a way due to their relative powerlessness in the present healthcare structure. Powerlessness results in the individual internalising feelings of defencelessness against the person or the structure whose superiority she/he fears. If the nurse is faced with unequal demands on their time, energy and personal resources, then symptoms of professional burnout could ensue, namely apathy, passive anger and callous and distancing approaches to patients and colleagues (Gould, 1990).

If nurse educators work in custodial ways, I suggest that students will demonstrate passivity and lack of assertiveness, which are outcomes of the process of becoming a nurse. Student experiences and their construction of their professional self become a direct consequence of power relationships in the context of healthcare. This limits their ability to be effective therapists and consequently the nursing care they deliver focuses on physical tasks, at the expense of establishing and maintaining therapeutic relationships with patients. For students to remain responsive to mentor's wishes, they must resist the values of self-authenticity. If students adhere to traditional educational methods and emulate the stereotype, their authentic selves go underground. Many students observe the stereotypical nursing behaviours in their mentors, who serve as role models for how nurses in this culture should act. As part of the socialisation process it may become apparent to students what behaviour nurses want to hear, and what can and cannot be said in order to be able to fit with the norms of nursing and thus belong. As students modify their behaviour in order to meet the demands of their professional self they begin to lose their authentic self and thus lose their voices. This means that often they are incapable of verbally expressing their authentic thoughts and feelings due to fear of reprisal.

Relationships between students and patients are an integral part of the socialisation process and nursing is stereotypically perceived to be a person-centred profession (Reed, 1992 and Bjork, 1995). However, many students witnessed scenarios that challenged this and they were aware that in some situations they consciously chose to act in a manner which they knew would have negative consequences for patients. Students who represented all four branches of nursing in the UK and who participated in my study, all started the course with a moral awareness of what was 'right' and 'wrong' (Reeve, 2000). They were able to articulate their shock and discomfort at witnessing nursing actions that placed patients in a vulnerable and precarious position. For instance, Susan was involved in a scenario where a learning disability client, named Heather, asked a staff nurse for some money. The staff nurse refused. Susan went on to tell me:

> I felt that it was Heather's money and that she was a grown woman who came across as knowing what she wanted. I felt she was being treated like a child just because she had a learning disability. If the staff nurse had just given Heather the money she needed and not even asked what Heather intended to buy, this incident wouldn't have happened.

Events such as this, which were mainly subtle in nature, left students experiencing moral distress. They experienced a conflict between an ideal image of the nurse they wanted to be and the type of nurse they were becoming. The effect of the process of becoming a nurse may have been a result of the fracturing of the self-esteem that these students experienced from the beginning of the course, which resulted in an inability to act in a beneficial and therapeutic manner towards patients.

Unfortunately, by the end of the course, students mainly appeared to be numb to the moral dilemmas facing them in their everyday practice. When interviewing Sally, who was at the end of her course, my fieldnotes described how I felt perturbed by her justifications that everything was 'just fine'. When reminding her of her earlier experiences of the course, where she expressed dilemmas concerning her role as a patient advocate, she replied:

> Oh, but you just have to fit in and get on with the work really. The patients don't mind, so long as they get treated, that's all they're bothered about. Honestly, everything's fine.

It was this student who was the most positive about how she felt as a prospective nurse, and throughout the interview she portrayed herself as having a healthy self-esteem. She liked herself as a nurse and felt it easy to communicate with staff, colleagues and patients, yet at the same time it also appeared that she was ambivalent in her thinking towards the way in which patients, staff and herself were treated. She felt nurses were bitchy, but this was OK as she 'didn't let it bother her'. This felt as if it was a testimony to her convictions about her current and future role, in which her interpretations of nursing were continually affirmed to her by the social system she now actively participated in.

The power of the socialisation process transformed them into stereotypical nurses of the context from they were educated. The authentic self bears the brunt of individual's reactions to experiences and as a consequence of the self being inherently evaluational, once students internalise the negative aspects of their professional self, it is imposed on the authentic self and thus becomes more resistant to change. This means that students and nurses work in ways that maintain the *status quo* and in relation to the concept of the therapeutic self means that this will be minimal. Evidence suggests that students and nurses often resist engaging in meaningful relationships with patients. I provide examples of student and nurse–patient interactions that are task-oriented, superficial and routine (Reeve, 2000). For instance, Peter, a student in the second week of his clinical practice who had not worked in healthcare prior to this, said:

> Great, last week I was practising basic skills; I removed a venflon, cared for pacemaker sites, took some obs and recorded them. Then I attended endoscopy with a patient for OGD; there wasn't any evidence of any root of referred pain apparent, though it was useful in discounting many possibilities like ulcers in the duodenum etc. I had a good chance to practice; I removed a CVP line, carried out an ECG, and attached cardiac monitors. I'm responsible for half of the ward; I monitored patients throughout the day, attended ward rounds, kept all records, handed over in the evening. During the ward round, though, I discovered a patient in the process of a MI. He was virtually asymptomatic but we gave him IV frusemide, oxygen and then we rushed him to CCU for thrombolysis. He was struggling and crying out at its peak. Diamorph, Isoket and Co-codamol provided some relief.

Apparent in this narrative was that Peter understood his role in terms of diagnosing and managing clinical conditions but that he had a low sense of empathy for the patient involved in this scenario. It is significant that he did not mention the use of communication skills such as reassuring the patient or 'being there'.

Reluctance to be self-aware and to attempt to develop interpersonal relationships is usual for people with low self-esteem (Reeve, 2000). Frequently, students talked about the technical parts of the job and ascribed high status to them. Dialogues that asserted the power of the techno-rationalist approach in the construction of the professional self were easily identifiable. By using technical speak, students were affirming their identification with the medical model and thus the authority this conferred on them as would-be nurses. As the course progressed, they became less willing to participate in the invisible roles of nursing, such as talking and listening, as quite simply they did not result in the same perceived gains as technical work. It is suggested that, as communication activities are difficult, if not impossible, to isolate and measure (Reeve, 2000), then little attention is paid to them.

Subjugation of communicative aspects of nursing practice was not a new finding and previous work has found that pre-registration diploma students are more interested in technically orientated tasks and are socialised to provide the traditional pattern of care (Hawthorne & Yurkovich, 1994). The biomedical model, with its focus on the patient's body, was the dominant framework students used to deliver their nursing care. Reliance on this model also explains the need to be competent with the technical aspects of nursing at the expense of patient-centred activities such as listening and information giving (May, 1990; Jarrett & Payne, 1995). Turner (1987), Emke (1992) and King (1992) agree with this and suggest that the technical aspects of healthcare take over the subjective aspects when a biomedical model is used.

Students in my study developed their sense of 'professional self' by involving themselves with the highly visible activities of being involved with technology. This is at the expense of communicating with patients, where their authentic self will have to come to the fore. The typical working day promotes the subjugation of the therapeutic self as interpersonal activities are confined to a fraction of the day, with the majority of time being taken up by physical care (Morrison & Burnard, 1997). Often, communicating with patients and sharing a sense of self can be seen as a 'luxury' or an 'extra' (Yam & Rossiter, 2000).

The organisation of nursing work meant that students soon assimilated that interpersonal skills were ascribed a low status by nurses and it was students, auxiliaries or healthcare assistants who were typically left to fulfil this role. Many students felt unsupported in this aspect of their learning and found it difficult to 'deal with' the emotional demands that it sometimes placed on them. Booth et al. (1996) and Reynolds et al. (2000) have highlighted the role of inadequate social support and support structures to deal with emotional distress as a barrier to effective communication. Yam and Rossiter (2000) suggest that improvements in colleague support could contribute to effective communication, compliance and satisfaction in healthcare.

It is not only the organisation of nursing work that limits the use of therapeutic self. As has been evident from the previous discussion, it is the psychological internalisation of nursing norms that has the most powerful effect. As self-esteem is the main predictor of behaviour (Bandura, 1995), those with low self-esteem are likely to adopt defensiveness as a strategy when dealing with the emotional labour of nursing (Smith, 1992). Emotional disengagement follows and thus the use of self becomes limited. Withdrawal and refusal to participate in activities where failure is predicted is characteristic of low self-esteem (Reeve, 2000). Effective interpersonal skills may result in 'getting involved' and may open floodgates to problems with which students and nurses are unable to cope. For individuals with low self-esteem, being placed in situations where they will be seen to be vulnerable as a result of too many demands on the self would be better avoided. The nurse educator in the clinical setting should be mindful of these negative effects, not only upon the student but also for her/himself. An example of the inability to cope with the emotional role can be seen in Karen's narrative:

> I thought he was absolutely disgusting. He was horrible. He shouldn't have done it, and I think he did it just to draw attention to himself. I've never seen a man naked other than my husband ... I just keep avoiding him now. I've asked if I can work within another team and I can't wait for him to be discharged. I spoke to my mentor about it because I don't know whether I should be feeling like this, but she said he was disgusting as well. He's still trying to get my attention and keeps trying to say 'hello' but I just ignore him.

In this instance, Karen and her mentor seem to be finding it difficult to relate to the patient as an individual. It may be that by vilifying the patient, the student can legitimately vent her/his rage and the hatred of the situation they find themselves in. Alternatively, as it appears through discussion with the student, the vilification of the patient may be a direct result of an awareness of the student's own inadequacies in dealing with the situation. For this student, the patient was the first male, other than her husband, that she had seen naked. Clearly she felt unprepared to deal with the intimacies of nursing care the role often necessitates. By placing disgust and blame onto the patient, the student is denying that it is 'her problem' – an attitude which is further confirmed by the support of her mentor's actions. Logically, by developing this stance, when the patient 'goes away' – that is, when he/she dies or is discharged – then the problem goes away. Unfortunately, for the patient, this is rarely the case. The nurse's inability to act therapeutically remains and so the next patient bears the brunt. The actual act of care giving and the emotional toll this may bring may actually jeopardise authenticity, as it is simply too much for the student and nurse to bear.

When looking at transforming nursing practice, nurse educators should take into account changes in the wider social and political nursing context. It is the unique perception of these events, then, which will help form the idea of the kind of student and nurse an individual is. Students and nurses with a healthy sense of self will perceive the many contextual changes as beneficial challenges and embrace a proactive stance. This is because they are the ones who are more likely to exert a degree of personal and professional agency. For those with a lower sense of self, it is likely that the challenging realities of nursing place heavy pressures on them and it is these people who are likely to be undermined by them. Students and nurses with a lower sense of self may lack the personal resources to cope effectively with changing environments and consequently experience deterious effects of a low sense of self.

The process of becoming a nurse may have a negative effect on the individual's self-esteem and would therefore be a hard price to pay in order to gain professional status. The educational implications of these findings are that students need from their mentors encouragement, validation and support for making their voices heard. They need the educational opportunities to be able to do so. Models where nurses simply instruct, handing the knowledge down to be mastered, will do little to support student voices. Students need opportunities, often in smaller groups, to present their ideas in a context where they will be listened to, heard and understood. Authoritarian teaching styles that provide knowledge in a uni-directional direction rob students of their own ideas and creativity. If educators transform their practice in order to build on student experiences, rather than rigid adherence to particular techniques and academic content, students will become engaged in the learning process. During this process it may be that their voices, and those of their patients, are heard.

References

Alavi, C. & Cattoni, J. (1995) 'Good nurse, bad nurse …'. *Journal of Advanced Nursing*, **21** (2), 344–9.
Andersson, E.P. (1993) 'The perceptions of student nurses and their perceptions of professional nursing during the nurse training programme'. *Journal of Advanced Nursing*, **18** (5), 808–815.

Arthur, D. (1992) 'Measuring the professional self-concept of nurses: a critical review'. *Journal of Advanced Nursing*, **17** (6), 712–19.

Arthur, D. & Thorne, S. (1998) 'Professional self-concept of nurses: a comparative study of four strata of nursing students in a Canadian university'. *Nurse Education Today*, **18** (5), 380–88.

Bandura, A. (1995) *Self-Efficacy in Changing Societies*. Cambridge: Cambridge University Press.

Barber, P. (1993) 'Developing the "person" of the professional carer' in Hinchcliff, S.M., Norman, S.E. & Schober, J.E. (eds). *Nursing Practice and Health Care*, 2nd edn. London: Edward Arnold. p. 344–73.

Bjork, I.I. (1995) 'Neglected conflicts in the discipline of nursing: perceptions of the importance and value of practical skill'. *Journal of Advanced Nursing*, **22** (1), 6–12.

Bloom, A. (1987) *The Closing of the American Mind*. Harmondsworth: Penguin.

Booth, K., Maguire, P.M., Butterworth, T. & Hillier, V. (1996) 'Perceived Professional Support and the use of Blocking Behaviours by Hospice Nurses'. *Journal of Advanced Nursing*, **24** (3), 522–7.

Briant, S. & Freshwater, D. (1998) 'Exploring Mutuality within the Nurse–Patient Relationship'. *British Journal of Nursing*, **7** (4), 204–211.

Bullivent, D. (1998) 'Crisis in nursing: An investigation into the reason for lack of interest in NHS nursing as a career'. Unpublished MSc Dissertation. University of Plymouth.

Bunkers, S.J. (1992) 'A strategy for staff development: self-care and self-esteem as necessary partners'. *Clinical Nurse Specialist*, **6** (3), 154–9.

Carson, J., Fagin, L., Brown, D., Leary, J. & Bartlett, H. (1997) 'Self-esteem in mental health nurses: its relationship to stress, coping and burnout'. *Nursing Times Research*, **2** (5), 361–70.

Cialdini, R.B., Wosinska, W., Barrett, D.W. & Gornik-Durose, M. (1999) 'Compliance with a request in two cultures: the differential influence of social proof and commitment/consistency on collectivists and individualists'. *Personality and Social Psychology Bulletin*, **25** (10), 1242–53.

Cook, S. (1999) 'The self in self-awareness'. *Journal of Advanced Nursing*, **29** (6), 1291–9.

Du Toit, D. (1995) 'A sociological analysis of the extent and influence of professional socialisation on the development of a nursing identity among nursing students at two universities in Brisbane, Australia'. *Journal of Advanced Nursing*, **21** (1), 164–71.

Emke, I. (1992) 'Medical authority and its discontents: a case of organised non-compliance'. *Critical Sociology*, **19** (3), 57–80.

Freshwater, D. (2000) 'Cross Currents: Against Cultural Narration'. *Journal of Advanced Nursing*, **32** (2), 481–4.

Freshwater, D. (1998). 'Transformatory learning in nurse education'. Unpublished PhD thesis. University of Nottingham.

Gould, D.I. (1990) 'Empathy: a review of the literature with suggestions for an alternative research strategy'. *Journal of Advanced Nursing*, **15** (10), 1167–74.

Hawthorne, D.L. & Yurkovich, N.Y. (1994) 'Caring: the raison d'etre of the professional nurse'. *The Canadian Journal of Nursing Administration*, **7** (4), 35–55.

Higgs, J. & Titchen, A. (eds) (2001) *Professional Practice in Health, Education and the Creative Arts*. Oxford: Blackwell Science.

Hogg, M.A. & Abrams, D. (1990) 'Social motivation, self-esteem and social identity' in Abrams, D. & Hogg, M.A. (eds). *Social Identity Theory: constructive and critical advances*. New York: Springer-Verlag. p. 28–47.

Jarrett, N. & Payne, S. (1995) 'A selective review of the literature on nurse–patient communication: has the patient's contribution been neglected?' *Journal of Advanced Nursing*, **22** (1), 72–8.

King, C.R. (1992) 'The ideological and technological shaping of motherhood'. *Women and Health*, **19** (2/3), 1–12.

McMahon, R. & Pearson, A. (eds) (1998) *Nursing as Therapy*, 2nd edn. Cheltenham: Stanley Thornes.

May, C. (1990) 'Research on nurse–patient relationships: problems of theory, problems of practice'. *Journal of Advanced Nursing*, **15** (3), 307–315.

Meeres, S.L. & Grant, P.R. (1999) 'Enhancing collective and personal self-esteem through differentiation: Further exploration of Hinkle and Brown's taxonomy'. *British Journal of Social Psychology*, **38** (1), 21–34.

Meissner, J. (1986) 'Nurses: are we eating our young?' *Nursing*, **16** (3), 51–3.

Morrison, P. & Burnard, P. (1997) *Caring and Communicating: The interpersonal relationship in nursing*. Basingstoke: Macmillan.

Mozingo, J., Thomas, S. & Brooks, E. (1995) 'Factors associated with perceived competency levels of graduating seniors in a baccalaureate nursing program'. *Journal of Nursing Education*, **34** (3), 115–22.

Olsen, J.K. (1995) 'Relationships between nurse expressed empathy, patient perceived empathy and patient distress'. *Image*, **27** (4), 317–22.

Randle, J. (2001) 'Past caring? The influence of technology'. *Nurse Education in Practice*, **1**, 157–65.

Reed, I. (1992) 'Individualised nursing care: some implications'. *Journal of Clinical Nursing*, **1** (1), 7–12.

Reeve, J. (2000) 'Past Caring?: A longitudinal study of the modes of change in the professional self-concept and global self-concepts of students undertaking a three-year diploma in nursing course'. Unpublished PhD dissertation. University of Nottingham.

Reynolds, W. & Scott, P. (2000) 'Do nurses and other professional helpers normally display much empathy?' *Journal of Advanced Nursing*, **31** (1), 226–34.

Reynolds, W., Scott, P. & Austin, W. (2000) 'Nursing, empathy and perception of the moral'. *Journal of Advanced Nursing*, **32** (1), 235–42.

Rogers, C. R. (1951) *Client-centred Therapy*. Boston: Houghton Mifflin.

Smith, P. (1992) *The Emotional Labour of Nursing – How Nurses Care*. Macmillan. Basingstoke.

Spouse, J. (1996) 'The effective mentor: a model for student centred learning in clinical practice'. *Nursing Times Research*, **11** (2), 120–33.

Terry, D.J., Hogg, M.A. & White, K.M. (1999) 'The theory of planned behaviour: Self-identity and group norms'. *British Journal of Social Psychology*, **38** (3), 225–44.

Turner, B. (1987) *Medical Power and Social Knowledge*. Sage: London.

Ulrich, Y.C. (1996) 'The relational self: views from feminism on development and caring'. *Issues in Mental Health Nursing*, **17** (4), 369–80.

White, E. (1996) 'Clinical supervision and Project 2000. The identification of some substantive issues'. *Nursing Times Research*, **1** (2), 102–111.

Yam, B.M.C. & Rossiter, J.C. (2000) 'Caring in nursing: perceptions of Hong Kong nurses'. *Journal of Clinical Nursing*, **9** (2), 293–302.

6 Aesthetic Ways in Day-to-day Nursing

Marilyn E. Parker

Good Morning I say to you, as I hold your hand and
smile with you, hoping to melt away all barriers,
hoping to bridge our spirits, to care, to nurture and
together soar like eagles over the day's challenges,
because I am your nurse.

(Libby, 1992)

This reflection by a nurse on her practice reminds us of the connections among the deeply held values of nursing, and aesthetic knowing and expression in nursing. Aesthetic expression in nursing can be created by exploring, understanding, appreciating and reflecting links of caring, aesthetic knowing and art. Such expressions, developed uniquely by each nurse, nurture continuing development of the person and nurse, and of relationships with others and the environment.

This chapter focuses on aesthetic knowing and expression as essential components of the discipline and profession of nursing. Included are aesthetic expressions of nurses' reflecting on their practice. Workshop formats have been developed and used for nurturing aesthetic knowing and expression, and are described. Assignments in undergraduate and graduate nursing courses in which students are encouraged to explore and create aesthetic expressions are offered as illustrations of teaching and learning for therapeutic nursing.

Preparing this chapter has offered opportunity to continue a personal path of discovery; reviewing earlier research and writing, I have reflected on my current work and added experiences from recent workshops and classroom sessions. With the emphasis on nurse education and ways of being teacher/learner, this chapter includes examples of developing caring ways to facilitate learning to know self and express self in nursing. Attention is given to creating environments conducive to such continuing growth.

Aiming to explore and share ways of teaching and learning, this chapter addresses the importance of knowing self and developing ways to continue to grow in this essential knowing. Knowing self requires learning ways to practice caring for self. In considering nurse as therapist, this chapter contributes ways for using self in nursing to facilitate mutually nurturing relational situations. These aspects of knowing, being and doing are interdependent, integrated and very practical; knowing and caring for self are requisite for using one's self in helpful ways as nurse. Hence the guiding concepts for the following work include ways of knowing in nursing, with special focus on overarching patterns of aesthetic knowing in nursing.

Setting the stage: an overview of essential nursing values and concepts of aesthetics and art in nursing

As a discipline of knowledge and unique professional practice, the essential value of respect for person is the basis of all that is truly nursing. Respect for person is lived uniquely in each nursing relationship through caring in nursing (Parker, 1994a; Parker & Barry, 1999). A prerequisite for nursing practice grounded in respect and caring is knowing and appreciating the innate and constant goodness of self and others and nurturing this goodness through relationships of practice. Multiple ways of knowing are used in the ongoing search to create and understand nursing based on respect and caring. While the explicit conception of nursing held by a nurse is the lens that specifies and guides the content and action of nursing, aesthetic ways of knowing have been found to be useful for exploring nursing as creative, unique and dynamic.

Caring is an essential nursing value. Caring, according to Mayeroff (1971), is helping the other grow. Major ingredients of caring are knowing, patience, honesty, trust, humility, hope, courage and alternating rhythms (Mayeroff, 1971). The work of this philosopher and author has formed the basis of understanding caring for many of the helping professions, including nursing. Nursing scholars since the time of Nightingale have centered their work on concepts of caring in nursing (Parker, 2001). Nursing philosopher Sr. Simone Roach states that caring is the human mode of being and that 'caring is the most authentic criterion of humanness' (1987: 2). Caring, while not unique to nursing, is unique in nursing and is expressed as compassion, competence, confidence, conscience and commitment (Roach, 1987).

Boykin and Schoenhofer (1993; 2001) assert that all persons are caring. These authors describe personhood as the process of living and uniquely expressing caring. Personhood is enhanced through participation in nurturing relationships, particularly in nursing relationships. Hence 'the unique focus of nursing is nurturing persons living caring and growing in caring' (Boykin & Schoenhofer, 1993: 21). Watson (1999; 2001) asserts that caring is the core, or essence, of nursing and sets forth concepts of clinical caritas and caritas processes. Transpersonal caring relationships are central to her work and are expressed in caring moments and caring occasions. Other nursing philosophers and theorists have set forth concepts of caring in nursing for practice, scholarship, education and organization (Benner & Wrubel, 1989; Gaut, 1984; Leininger, 1991; Newman, 1994; Ray, 2000; Swanson, 1993).

Concepts of aesthetics and art

As the philosophy of the beautiful, aesthetics is focused on beauty, the creating, knowing and appreciating the beautiful. As a branch of philosophy, aesthetics addresses a range of problems about our understanding of art, creativity and goodness in art, including concepts we use in thinking and speaking about art (Beardsley, 1966; Kennick, 1979). The ways we think and speak about, and ways we engage with art has been influenced by classic and modern philosophers and artists. Tolstoy (1930) wrote that art advances human wellbeing by enhancing unity and facilitating communication. The processes of creating art are essential to the artist. The act of creating, not the artistic product, is of primary interest to the artist (Richards, 1962; Tomas, 1968; Berensohn, 1972). Art encourages aesthetic experience through personal encounter with the art object (Beardsley, 1969).

Kazanis (1992) describes a new paradigm of art as compassionate action with art being understood within all of life. Art is experience, skill and form, using ability for aesthetic expression. Art is work exhibiting creativity. Art must be recognized as not only an object but as a process that enhances communication, unity and wellbeing. Moore (1992) suggests that by living artfully we can let day-to-day living bring us into reflection and lead us to new expression. Indeed, living and practicing aesthetically can be taught and learned and can therefore advance creative and effective communication and interconnections, bringing healing for self and others.

Historically, there was no separation between the person and the art (Dooling, 1979). The craft guilds preceded our professions; going back to the ideals of these groups may be helpful as we consider aesthetics and art. A particular art form was a paradigm of the whole activity of the person. The person was known as person making or doing, both grounded in contemplation, whether he/she be painter, weaver, potter or poet. Coomaraswamy (1956) maintains that creativity must not be considered lightly, and that ideas for art and creativity are gifts of Spirit, not to be confused with talents. Further, the artist or creator is servant of what he or she makes or does. The artist receives the new and unique form, in service to the art, not as its owner. Aesthetics and art as form that expresses real, practical and sensuous experience is an open mystery (Kazanis, 1992).

Aesthetics and art in nursing

Nursing as art has a secure place in popular descriptions of nursing. Since the work of Carper (1975), perspectives on aesthetics and art in nursing have been the focus of nursing scholars (Aita, 1990; Boykin et al., 1998; Diekelmann, 1990; Donohue, 1985; Heighley & Ferentz, 1988; Lange, 1990; LeVasseur, 1999; Oiler, 1983; Parker & Schoenhofer, 1990; Schoenhofer, 1989; Smith, 1992). Various art forms have been used to enhance understanding nurses and their prac-tice (Gordon, 1997; Locsin, 1998; Wagner, 2000). Although there is scholarly interest in these areas for nursing education and practice, no nursing theory or philosophy has emerged to lead the development of aesthetics and art in nursing. However, several reports of exploration of art and aesthetics in nursing that have recently appeared in the literature include the following: Johnson's (1994) analysis of works of 41 nursing authors between 1860 and 1992 revealed five distinct concepts that were identified as art:

1   Grasping meaning in encounters with patients.
2   Making meaningful connections with patients.
3   Performing nursing skillfully.
4   Determining appropriate course of nursing action.
5   Morally conducting nursing practice.

Hampton (1994) analyzed the concept of expertise as the essence of nursing art. Wainwright (2000) explored art and aesthetics of nursing, including a critique of Carper's work, and concluded that nursing may be a legitimate focus of aesthetic expression and that good nursing practice may be described as having aesthetic quality.

Carper (1975; 1978) brought the concepts of aesthetics and aesthetic knowing in nursing to the structure of the discipline and to nurse education. Four patterns of knowing in nursing were identified from an analysis of the literature. Carper (1975; 1978) described these as:

- empirics, the science of nursing;
- esthetics, the art of nursing;
- the component of a personal knowledge in nursing; and
- ethics, the component of moral knowledge.

In describing aesthetics as the art of nursing, Carper acknowledges that this is a limited meaning and has left a way open for developing and using the concept of nursing aesthetics as more than either nursing arts or the use of art in nursing.

Boykin et al. (1994) examined philosophical literature on aesthetics and reflected on their personal experiences of aesthetic knowing in nursing practice and education. Following a review of Carper's work, these authors described a broader and more inclusive understanding of aesthetic knowing in nursing. This conception holds that aesthetic knowing in nursing is creating and expressing nursing, and includes the appreciation of experience through encounter with art (Boykin et al., 1994).

The *experience* of aesthetic knowing in nursing is primary. Further, each experience of creating, expressing and appreciating is simultaneously unique and universal, is not only new but also connected with other similar experiences (Boykin et al., 1994). This can be illustrated through reflecting on an experience; describing special attributes of that experience; recognizing relations with elements of other experiences; and then using reflections on these several nursing experiences to inform future nursing practice. While a full range of expert knowing can inform nursing practice, the actual experiences of nursing are not the result of design or planning and the outcome of nursing cannot be predicted. Instead, 'Nursing aesthetics is in the mutually appreciated experience of nursing, rather than in the product of nursing' (Boykin et al., 1994: 159).

Empirics, ethics and personal knowing are not sufficient for full understanding of nursing. Aesthetic knowing is used to unify, transform and communicate all other ways of knowing in nursing. Nursing practice is a dynamic, artistic process that is continually unfolding, and thus is an ongoing aesthetic experience. Active awareness and use of aesthetic knowing is the highest form of knowing in nursing. Aesthetic expression manifests knowing in nursing and is at once being, doing and making, so that our reflections, visions, inner experiences and remembered connections are brought forth and created as presence. The expression is new and unique for the one creating and also for those viewing or participating in the art. Through reflection and aesthetic expression we gain insight and make real our knowing, and then we view, share, listen and hear from our art and continue to learn.

Each of us is artist when we live as fully, openly and faithfully as we can. As person and as nurse, we can live authentically, offer genuine presence, overcome separateness and remember wholeness. The nurse artist values the unique individual subjective experience and often does not foresee what will result from nursing. The nurse artist has heightened awareness, seeking mutuality of caring and harmony of action (Parker, 1992). Therefore, forms of nursing as art are always new, yet they seem timeless, 'the nurse artist experiences energy for her/his work and enhanced wellbeing in her/his life' (1992: 34).

Below is a summary to date of my own and others' current research in this area:

* Art and aesthetic expressions unite us and contribute to our wholeness. They are essential means of communication and move all of us toward increased wellbeing.
* Experiences with art and with aesthetic expression surpass the senses and are about truth and reality rather than emotion. Aesthetic knowing is more than and different from other kinds of knowing. Aesthetic knowing provides an umbrella of understanding of empirical, ethical and personal knowing.
* Artistic processes and the art itself are central to thinking about aesthetics. Both expressions and experience are essential to aesthetics and aesthetic knowing in nursing. The expressions and experiences of nursing are specific, unique and whole acts of creation. The creating, not the object created, is primary. Outcomes cannot be predicted.
* The artist as creator is fully present, authentic and open to receive and to do. In nursing at its best, the nurse does not act and react with superficial, expected or predicted behavior. The nurse responds from more than the intention of the person as nurse. The nursing response gives up the known to receive that which is central and unknown and a creative nursing response is offered.
* Nursing, as art and as aesthetic expression, gives the nurse opportunity to express her/himself in unique ways from within and from beyond the self. Aesthetic expressions are always new, personal and subjective, and therefore

seem difficult to describe. The expressions cannot be generalized, but can serve to inform future practice.

Creating aesthetic expressions in nursing

Linking concepts of aesthetics, aesthetic knowing and nursing values provides structure and process for creating aesthetic expressions of nursing. Persons who choose to express their nursing by artistic means seek to know their own unique meaning of nursing and ways their nursing is lived. These aesthetic expressions have both unique and universal attributes; they can bring to light goodness and full humanness of persons in nursing situations. Creative authentic ways of relating with self, others and the environment are both reflected and encouraged.

Creating paths of aesthetic expression may also be chosen or developed by persons pursuing aesthetic ways in day-to-day life and in their nursing. Particular disciplines or patterns of activities may be described as having aesthetic qualities and may include making and doing art (yoga, meditation, reflective practice exercises, journaling, playing a musical instrument, dancing, caring for self). These activities may be developed into aesthetic paths that integrate aesthetic knowing and caring and serve to enhance the wellbeing of the person as person and person as nurse. Each unique caring path may use and provide art to nurture personal strength, discipline, endurance, grace and beauty. The person is thus gently moved toward an increasingly vital, caring-filled life, rich in value and meaning, balanced with quiet reflection and creative expression, and with attention to natural interconnections and openness to discovery.

Creating the setting for aesthetic expression in nursing education, practice and scholarship: illustrations

Some environmental elements essential to encouraging aesthetic expression are described in sections to follow. Other environmental considerations include a comfortable space (clean, warm, uncluttered and uncrowded) and enough time to work without a sense of feeling rushed. Comfortable clothing is important. Chairs and the needed workspace should be inviting and supportive. The tone set by the teacher/facilitator should be one of acceptance, hope, expectancy, compassion and confidence, recognizing each person as worthy of respect for the gifts each brings and offers to the experience. This genuine tone can readily be welcomed and joined in by the other participants.

Opportunities for aesthetic expression as a one-time event or paths of aesthetic expression may be created and lived in the context of caring community. Attributes of such a community include a safe, comfortable place in which self and others are honored and where listening and sharing contribute to nurturing growth of all (Parker & Barry, 1999). Mayeroff (1971) describes communities of integrity in which caring ingredients are integrated: knowing, patience, honesty, hope and courage. The experience of developing and following a path of aesthetic expression within such a community may be expected to lead to a sense of being connected and complete, beautiful and boundless, sharing love, courage and hope (further reading in this area include Boykin (1994); Boykin & Parker (1997; Parker et al. (2000); and Applebaum, (2000)).

The workshop format

A workshop format has been developed and used to explore rituals and art forms facilitating experiences of aesthetic expression. Use of this format may lead to expressions of reflections on nursing or may be developed into ongoing paths of aesthetic expression for individual enrichment. Examples are workshops in motion and dance, watercolor, mindful meditation, yoga and Tai Chi. These workshops often include a quiet time and place for reflection and expression. Art seems to link inner being and outer world, reminding us of connections and making us more aware and alive. Remembering our wholeness and our interconnection with our experiences and each other are desired themes.

The following is a description of a clay workshop that includes perspectives from a formerly published work (Parker, 1994b). A similar format can be employed regardless of the medium of clay, drawing or writing that is central to the experience (see Figure 6.1).

Introduction to the clay workshop

The environment should be safe and comfortable, without crowding and distraction. Caring environments support contemplation and reflection and contemplation. For example, soft, gentle instrumental music will form a background intended to provide for ease and support reflection and expression. Music should be free of specific cultural reference and words that might invite former experiences.

> - Personal growth takes place in safe, comfortable places.
> - Each person is creative.
> - Creating art leads to inner knowing places.
> - The creative process is healing, connecting us with all beings.
> - Each culture has a heritage of art.
> - The play of children is often artistic.
> - Expressions of caring are evident in most ceremony and ritual.
> - Caring is evident in making useful and beautiful objects.
> - Mindfulness of our self, our body, our wholeness brings us to joining with the clay.

Figure 6.1   *Using art to access creative therapeutic potential*

Brief instruction about working with clay is offered to increase ease of participants. Some ways of joining with the clay are described, including simple techniques of opening, circling, pinching and use of fingers, elbows and knees. Ways to choose and prepare clay and select various tools are described. Simple demonstrations and examples may be offered.

Meditation and reflection

Meditations, poems written by Progoff (1971a; 1971b), have been used to help as participants enter a quiet, deep place where inner knowing is available. Progoff (1971a) suggests that meditation can bring us to a place within ourselves so we can reach beyond ourselves, 'freeing ourselves to respond to our own rhythms and move in directions that feel right to us' (1971a: 13). Thus the results of our finding ways to meditate and reflect can be the same for us as the fish finding his way in the water. The fish does what is natural and learns to swim. We do what comes natural to us and find our way to be creative and grow. An example of a Progoff entrance *meditation* follows:

The Center Point Within Me

1. We are resting,
    Physically quiet,
    Breath and body
    In gentle harmony
    Holding the stillness within.

2. Holding the stillness within,
    Thoughts fit into place.
    No longer spinning,
    They come together;
    No longer disputing,
    Our thoughts
    Are friendly with each other.
    The quality of wholeness
    Replaces
    The discord of the mind.

3. Mind and body
    Together,
    Thoughts and emotions
    Revolving around
    A single center point.
    Varied movements
    Actively churning
    Form a quiet center.
    A quiet center forms
    In their midst.

4. We feel the center of our Self
    The inner center of our Self,
    It is neither body
    Nor mind
    But a center point.
    Not this, not that,
    A single center point,
    The inner center of the Self.

5. In the midst of activity
    Soft, slow breathing
    Sets a balance.
    An inward stillness
    Becomes present.
    The center point within me
    Establishes itself.

6. For each of us it is so.
    A center point within
    Forms itself.
    A center point is present
    Not in space
    But in our being.

7. A center point within me.
    My whole attention
    At that center point,
    Present there in the stillness,
    In the stillness of the Self.

8. Through this center point
    We move inward,
    Inward and downward
    Through a single straight shaft.
    It is as though we go
    Deep into the earth,
    But within our Self.
    Through the center point within.
    We go inward,
    Deeper,
    Deeper inward.

9. My life
    Is like the shaft of a well.
    I go deep into it.
    The life of each of us
    Is a well.
    Its sources are deep,
    But it gives water on the surface.
    Now we go inward,

Moving through our center point,
Through our center point,
Deeply inward to explore
The infinities of our well.

10. Long enough
    We have been on the surface
    Of our life.
    Now we go inward,
    Moving through our center point
    Inward,
    Into the well of our Self,
    Deeply,
    Further inward
    Into the well of our Self.

11. We move away
    From the surface of things;
    We leave
    The circles of our thoughts,
    Our habits, our customs.
    All the shoulds
    And the oughts
    Of our life
    We leave behind.

12. We leave them on the surface
    While we go inward,
    Into the depth of our life
    Moving through the center point
    Into the well of our Self
    As deeply
    As fully
    As freely as we can.
    Through the center point
    Exploring the deep places.
    Exploring the deep places
    In the Silence … In the Silence

(Progoff, 1971b: 59–86)

Sharing aesthetic expressions

Following a time of working with the clay, participants are invited to share their experiences, their aesthetic expressions and hopes and dreams for the possible future of their work. One nursing student described the freedom she felt as she began to express her nursing reflections in drawing and then with the clay. The sculpture of one nurse was named *Spirit Woman* and a poem describing the art object was also written. The nurse wrote that as she finished the object and the poem she was energized:

I did it? I listened to me and found a part that was lost. I felt such a sense of wonder at what my soul and hands could do together. I thought: ah, this was meant to be! I have much love in my life from others, what has been missing is my own spirit. I have been on a vision quest for many months. I have been struggling with: Where am I going? Who am I? What is my purpose in life? There must be more to life than this. I do not have these answers even now. What I do have is my *Spirit Woman*; I have found my spirit connection. Now I will not travel my roads alone. (Parker, 1994b: 140–43)

I find that I, too, am moved to write reflectively in response to my experience of working with clay:

> The clay, the pot, the person
> The potter, the nurse
> All being flows from the center.
> Person and pot are both vessels built from the inside
> with integrity as an acclaimed value of each. Both are
> living – some say clay dies in the fire, some say it
> becomes more alive. Is this true also of the person?
> I am nurse, I am with the inner person to respond to
> calls for help to be what he can be and for assistance
> to become that which he can become. The person and
> clay are as one. The clay depends on the person as the
> person depends on the clay. When I am with the clay,
> I center, the clay centers. The issues, problems, dreams,
> longings belong to the vessel, not to the potter or to the nurse.
> The clay is alive as we are alive, and the clay is
> willing to grow with us. We come to know the clay when
> we realize that, like us, it can move, stretch, take new
> forms, be acclaimed for its beauty and usefulness. And,
> we come to know the clay as we recognize that it seems
> to have limits. Like us, it can be pushed too far, stretched
> beyond its capacity to respond. Potters will advise to 'let
> the clay rest'. Its strength and flexibility is restored by
> resting. Like us, the clay has spirit, uniqueness and
> connections with the larger whole. The clay is living.
> The clay will let you know what it is and what it
> will become.

Alternatives for workshop format

Options for the workshop format include offering an invitation to reflect on therapeutic nursing values and then to write a story of nursing that reflects that value. The nurse is then encouraged to create an expression of the nursing situation using artistic means. Examples of therapeutic nursing values held most dear include: caring for persons the way I want my family members cared for; keeping my patients safe; and connection with those I nurse and with my colleagues. Frequently, nurses realize that their nursing values are the same as their values as person and that they are truly integrated as person and nurse, that is to say that nursing is a way of being.

The writing or telling of the nursing situation helps nurses remember that their closely held values and beliefs are integral to their day-to-day nursing and the doing and being of nursing is actually grounded in essential values. This knowing seems to elevate the view of nursing beyond the discrete facts and actions we often call nursing, to an understanding of the truth and beauty of nursing, the aesthetics of nursing. Creating an aesthetic expression is the next step in the workshop process.

Illustrations from academic courses

Use of aesthetic expression to teach nursing is based in part on research of the experience of nursing of the nurse artist. Findings demonstrated the nurse artist values unique individual nursing experiences and that reflecting on these experiences brings one to know the fullness of nursing (Parker, 1992). Aesthetic expression of nursing is built on knowing nursing as art and understanding that offering and perceiving aesthetic expressions of nursing leads to further appreciation of nursing by self and by others. Exploring and engaging in paths of aesthetic expression, activities that are nurturing of therapeutic self, are also recognized as experiences that may facilitate understanding and growth in self and understanding ways to nurture growth in others. The illustrations that follow are all examples of nursing students who offered their work as illustrations of course assignments; permission has been sought to reproduce.

The *Aesthetic Project and Scholarly Paper* assignment

The *Aesthetic Project and Scholarly Paper* is an assignment I have used in graduate and undergraduate nursing courses. The purpose of this assignment is to nurture scholarly understanding and experience of caring in nursing, combined with a theory of caring in nursing. Students are asked to reflect on a nursing situation, connect it with a theory of caring in nursing, express this in an aesthetic mode and describe the experience in a brief but scholarly paper. Aesthetic expressions may be in many forms: poetry, song, needlework, painting, posters or other means of artistic presentation. Each student presents his/her aesthetic project and scholarly paper to the class, followed by comments, discussion and questions. The last part of the paper is a self-evaluation of the experience, a grade for the project and rationale for the grade. Evaluation guidelines include attention to the following:

- Expression of the nursing situation as a story of the lived experience of caring in nursing.
- Connection of the nursing situation with a theory of caring in nursing.
- Effectiveness of the aesthetic expression of the nursing situation.
- Meaning of the project to student as person and as nurse.
- Potential impact of the project on contemporary nursing.
- Discovered insights or issues about caring in nursing.

Following are examples of student work for this assignment. The first is an aesthetic expression created following reflection on a nursing situation in which the patient died:

I'M FREE

Don't grieve for me, for now I'm free
I'm following the path God laid for me.
I took His hand when I heard Him call
I turned my back and left it all.
I could not stay another day
To laugh, to love, to work or play.
Tasks left undone must stay that way.
I found that peace at close of day.
If my parting has left a void,
Then fill it with remembered joy.
A friendship shared, a laugh, a kiss.
Ah, yes, these things I too will miss.
Be not burdened with times of sorrow
I wish you the sunshine of tomorrow.
My life's been full; I've savored much.
Good friends, good time, a loved one's touch.
Perhaps my time seemed all to brief,
Don't lengthen it now with undue grief.
Lift up your hearts and share with me,
I'm with God now, I've been set free.

Robin M. Magro

This is a nursing situation described by a student on reflection through art:

A week of diagnostic studies revealed a reality that Gregory was not expecting to confront. A virulent, cancerous lesion was consuming his physical shell, leaving a soul, raw and broken, to accept a premature imminent death. During his final days he suffered from hypertension and paralysis; he found comfort with the presence of his family and caregivers. Despite feelings of fear and despair, Gregory accepted that he was dying and on the evening of his death as he looked into death's eyes, I asked him to tell me of the one place on earth that would bring him peace and comfort. He described a tree where he would like to sprawl, breathe and listen to the sound of his beating heart. I held his hand and through our mind's eyes, we envisioned a river bank and focused on the trees: the twisted winding of their branches, the sound of the breeze against the leaves of their color laden foliage and the touch of the coarse bark against our backs.

This student used Watson's theory of nursing to describe more fully and understand the nursing situation, and drawings of trees in various settings to represent the nursing situation.

The *Caring for Self Project* assignment

The *Caring for Self Project* forms part of the same course and is based on the well documented understanding that nurses often care for others to the neglect of caring for self, and that growth can be encouraged by enhancing respect for self and providing special care for self. The assignment was inspired by the very popular course, *Caring For Self*, as a way to introduce students who might otherwise not have this experience. Each student is asked to choose and engage in a caring for self activity of his/her choice for one hour weekly. At the end of the semester, a one page paper is submitted that describes the activity, why the activity was selected, and a reflection on how this activity helped to nurture wholeness and wellbeing.

- The *Journaling* assignment in this course required a weekly entry of reflections, insights and ideas that form practice and the nursing literature; it also provides an opportunity for exploring nursing situations. Times for sharing with colleagues in class is arranged. Following is an example taken from a student journal:

> This is my last journal entry for this semester. At times I have had to force myself to think and reflect about my nursing. Today I presented my aesthetic project and I feel exhilarated. I think that everything we were trying to accomplish in this course finally came together for me. It is one thing to be able to talk and write on a subject, it is quite another to feel and live it. You said in the beginning of the semester that you wanted our journals to reflect growth. I'm not sure if you can determine if I grew from my writing, but I truly have. While developing my aesthetic project, everything clicked. I experienced an increase in my personal knowing while communicating my nursing situation aesthetically.
>
> Technology is an ever-present partner in our nursing world. We are expected to know machines, how they work, what all the bells and whistles mean and how to effectively incorporate all of that into our nursing. With the time constraints we all feel, when do we have time to tend to our patients ... we have to tend to the technology? As nurses we need to make that time, both for patients and for ourselves. In the ER we are surrounded by technology to do about everything for our patients except what I think they most often need – a warm smile, holding their hand, or a gentle nod that yes, someone is listening. On reflection, I have come to understand that I can provide caring for my patients through touch and a smile while I am also caring for them by using the machines. I hope I don't get caught up in attending only the technology again.

The *Caring for Self* academic course

Caring for Self, a three-credit academic course, was developed by Dr Eleanor Schuster, who has offered her syllabus and her experiences for publication in this chapter (personal communication, October 2000). The course is one in which students and faculty address personal mind/body/spirit connections as integral to healing and health. Each student is his/her own 'laboratory', learning to make choices that support personal wellbeing and that are relevant to nurturing the wellbeing of others. Topics of the course include content and experiences about energy and energy work, touch, centering, listening, celebrating life passages and honoring self. The required text is *The Artist's Way* by Julia Cameron (1992). *The Four-Fold Way* (Arien, 1993) and *Holistic Nursing: A Handbook for Practice* (Dossey, 2000) are recommended texts.

Assignments for this course include daily journaling and a weekly 'artists date', which is a weekly activity chosen and done by oneself, alone. Both are described in the Cameron text (1992). The journal is not submitted, but a paragraph describing the artist's date and its meaning to the student is submitted weekly. The student signs a contract agreeing to the assignments and submits a grade for self at the end of the course. Justification for the grade includes evidence of personal and professional growth, insights, readings, experiences and accomplishments, disappointments, mistakes, as well as goals and joys.

A study of students and faculty who completed two sections of the course during the first year it was taught was reported (Schuster, 1998). Fifty-seven graduate and undergraduate students and faculty evaluated the course at the conclusion of the course and after 6 months. Findings indicated an increased awareness of and respect for personal power; an ability to act with focus and deliberation on behalf of personal wellbeing; an increased clarity and depth of understanding of personal attributes and skills; adaptability of newfound insights to personal and professional roles; transferability of new knowledge to client, colleague and other relationships.

Evaluative comments of students include the following:

I love the morning pages (journaling) and plan to continue with this as part of my life. I have encountered many instances of 'synchronicity' and have found myself becoming freer in spirit and creative areas of my life. It was like I have let go of old things in my life that were holding me down and keeping me low. I feel as if I have been scratching with the chickens and now I am beginning to soar with the eagles. Things unfolded in my life as I wrote those pages. I found I was not as irritable as I used to be, because now I had an outlet.

The artist's dates were enriching to my life and made me aware that I need time for my own self because I am important. I always put others' interests first above mine. It is time to be a little crazy and extravagant for my own peace of mind. I will continue on the dates, not now for an assignment but for me, because I want to do so.

Reflecting on nursing practice

Purposes of reflection on practice include helping nurses increase their awareness and improve the quality of their practice (Johns & Freshwater, 1998). Nurses often are willing to share their reflections and in doing so may increase their colleagues' awareness and enhance quality of nursing care more widely. Aesthetic expressions of reflection on practice may emerge or be created and then shared. Nurses have shared their aesthetic expressions with clients and family members to advance understanding and validate shared experiences. Each such expression has potential for leading to deeper knowing and understanding by the nurse and by others who share the expression. *Nightingale Songs* (Parker & Schoenhofer, 1990) is an occasional publication designed for the purpose of sharing nurses' reflections on their practice. Many of the following reflections have been submitted to and published in *Nightingale Songs*.

Reflections and aesthetic expressions of those reflections have been used to teach students about reflective practice and about the wholeness and beauty of nursing (Cope & Parker, 1994). Each nurse or student who shares the illustration enters the situation and becomes an active participant. Through this sharing the connections of persons experiencing the situation in unique ways is evident. Thus the situation is often renewed, appreciated and continues to inform practice.

Nursing students are assisted to learn nursing through reflecting on a situation of their own nursing, a story of the lived experience of caring between the nurse and the client. Nursing students can also read and reflect on the nursing stories or aesthetic expressions of others in order to understand more fully and appreciate nursing. The following questions are used to teach reflection on nursing situations. The questions are designed to reflect the concept of nursing held by the nursing faculty at Florida Atlantic University (Philosophy, 1994).

Who is this person as caring person?
What are the unique hopes and dreams of this person?
What are the person's unique calls for nursing?
What are ranges of calls for nursing that can be understood through this nursing situation?
What are specific nursing responses of caring that may promote wholeness and well being of the person?

(Cope & Parker, 1994: 50)

The reader is invited to peruse the following aesthetic expressions by nurses written as reflections on their nursing practice, and to use these questions to gain understanding through aesthetic knowing of the nursing situation. This is the way the poems are used to teach nursing: students are assisted to envision coming to know the patient in the poem and to name calls for nursing that he/she experiences through the study of the situation. The student then creates and suggests nursing responses that may be called for in the situation. Each student is supported in this learning by the reminder that each nursing call and response is unique and is dependent on the client and nurse in the situation. Therefore, there may be as many perceived calls and created responses as there are students in the class.

Isolation Precautions

I

Some drive you deep
unto the coils of your self
not because of your being,
not because of your soul,
but because
of what you might give them
in return.
One of them was here.
Lady in white was here.
She had hopes for you.

She had wishes for you
and she gave you time.
But she was half in, half out,
isolation precautions,
The sign told all,
the reason for the masks and gowns,
and how you were
to be separated from them.

II

She wore boots over her shoes
so she won't have to pass the
broken paths you've trod.
The mask covered her mouth
to silence her asking.
She already knows you.
The goggles over her eyes
to blur your suffering
for she understood your hurt.
The gowns were donned
to keep you from being too near
her immaculate body.
There was no time, no hope,
no need for others to be close.
The gloves covered her hands
so she did not have to touch
your sore,
after all your end was near.

III

I was here
but I wore the boots
so I can trace your footsteps,
to where you've been
so I too can partake of
your journeys past
and guide you to where
you're going.
I wore the mask
so I can remember
that soothing sounds come
not only from my tongue
but also from my body
which shouts the louder.
I wore the cap on my head
to remember that you are human
as much as I am human.
I wore gloves
to remember that what touches you
are not my hands,

what touches you
is my soul.

(Madayag, 1993)

Anne

She stood transfixed
in disbelief
Her expression
filled with fear
wide eyes surveyed
the tiny babe.
As they filled up ...
and then a tear
spilled down her cheek.
As I opened the isolette,
'you can touch her hand'
I said.
Hesitantly, very hesitantly
her fingers touched lightly ...
A tiny hand grasped tightly.
She smiled through
the tears.
her name is 'Anne' she said.

(Drozdowicz, 1992)

Final Journey

Your eyes are watching God –
Focused on a place I have not been, and cannot go
But still, my job is to take you there.
If I do it well, I loose you
Yet, what else is left?
Hand in hand, we start on the road to eternity.
I stop, you go on
The caring never ends.

(Gulbrandsen, 1990)

Love is a Small Spoon

I took a tiny frame 93 years of age, (and much less in pounds) curled up in the same
position as in the womb, and I wonder, dear Lord ... what goes through her mind?

She's unable to speak, and so weak she can hardly move.
She DEPENDS on those around her to meet her needs.
She gets something to drink when I offer it, something to eat with I feed her.
Ah, yes, she DEPENDS, Lord, on those of us around her.

She's fortunate, this little lady, that those who tend to her needs really love her. I've been told she loves mashed potatoes and hates spinach … and told definitely to use a small spoon, please!
This frail frame, almost lost in the bed sheets, will only be with us for a short while … then she'll be back at the nursing home with those who know about small spoons and mashed potatoes.
But I still wonder what goes through her mind! Does she pray? Does she talk to you, Lord? She'll have to DEPEND on you, oh Lord, for you are around her more than anyone. I know she'll do fine … because you know all about mashed potatoes and small spoons, but more importantly.
You know how to nourish her and care for her, and give what she needs most!
All this reminds me dear Lord, of how I must DEPEND on YOU! For my lines and needs!
You feed me with your Eucharist and Your Scripture … (much better than mashed potatoes).

I thank you Lord, for feeding me when you choose … and not giving me spinach too often.
I thank you Lord, for allowing me just to be still … curled up under the sheets when I   need to rest … and waiting for you to 'move me'.
I thank you most of all Lord, for that loving touch … that knows the unique me so well,   that knows how to feed me with a small spoon!
I am truly grateful … Bless my 93-year-old patient, Lord. Bless me … (Oetting, 1991)

References

Aita, V. (1990) 'The art of nursing'. *Nurse Educator*, **15** (6), 24–8.
Applebaum, D. 2000 (ed.) 'The teacher' in *Parabola: Myth, Tradition, and the Search for Meaning*. **25** (3), 6–159.
Arien, A. (1993) *The Four-fold Way*. New York: HarperCollins.
Beardsley, M.C. (1966) 'On the creation of art'. *Journal of Aesthetics and Art Criticism*, **23**, 291–304.
Beardsley, M.C. (1969) *Asethetics: From Classical Greece to the Present*. New York: Macmillan.
Benner, P. & Wrubel, J. (1989) *The Primacy of Caring*. Menlo Park, CA: Addison Wesley.
Berensohn, P. (1972) *Finding One's Way with Clay*. New York: Simon & Schuster.
Boykin, A. (ed.) (1994) *Living the Caring-Based Program*. New York: National League for Nursing Press.
Boykin, A. & Parker, M. (1997) 'Illuminating spirituality in the classroom' in Sr. Roach, S. (ed.). *Caring from the Heart: The Convergence of Caring and Spirituality*. New York: Paulist Press. pp. 21–33.
Boykin, A., Parker, M. & Schoenhofer, S. (1994)'Aesthetic knowing grounded in an explicit conception of nursing'. *Nursing Science Quarterly*, **7** (4), 158–61.
Boykin, A., Parker, M. & Touhy, T. (1998) 'Discovering the beauty of older adults – Opening doors'. *Journal of Clinical Geropsychology*, **4** (3), 201–210.
Boykin, A. & Schoenhofer, S. (1993) *Nursing as Caring: A Model for Transforming Practice*. New York: National League for Nursing Press.
Boykin, A. & Schoenhofer, S. (2001) 'Nursing as caring' in Parker, M. *Nursing Theories and Nursing Practice*. Philadelphia: F.A. Davis. p. 391–409.
Cameron, J. (1992) *The Artist's Way*. New York: G.P. Putnam's Sons.

Carper, B. (1975) 'Fundamental patterns of knowing in nursing'. PhD dissertation. Teachers College, Columbia University, New York.

Carper, B. (1978) 'Fundamental patterns of knowing in nursing'. *Advances in Nursing Science*, **1** (1), 13–23.

Coomaraswamy, A.K. (1956) *Christian and Oriental Philosophy of Art*. New York: Dover Publications.

Cope, D. & Parker, M. (1994) 'The shared study of nursing' in Anne Boykin (ed.). *Living the Caring Based Program*. New York: National League for Nursing Press. p. 43–63.

Diekelmann, N. (1990) 'Nursing education: Caring, dialogue, and practice'. *Journal of Nursing Education*, **29** (7), 300–305.

Donohue, M. (1985) *Nursing: The Finest Art*. St. Louis: C.V. Mosby Co.

Dooling, D.M. (1979) *A Way of Working: The Spiritual Dimension of Craft*. New York: Parabola Books.

Dossey, B. (2000) *Holistic Nursing: A Handbook for Practice*. Gaithersberg, MD: Aspen Publishers, Inc.

Drozdowicz, C. (1992) 'Anne' in *Nightingale Songs*, **2** (3), 2, P.O. Box 057563, West Palm Beach, FL. 33405.

Gaut, D. (1984) 'A theoretic description of caring as action' in Leininger, M. (ed.) *Caring: The Essence of Nursing and Health*. Thorofare. NJ: Stack. p. 17–24.

Gordon, S. (1997) 'Using visual descriptions to explore nursing values over time'. *International Journal for Human Caring*, **1** (2), 16–21.

Gulbrandsen, M. (1990) 'Final Journey' in *Nightingale Songs*, **1** (2), 2, P.O. Box 057563, West Palm Beach, FL. 33405.

Hampton, D.C. (1994) 'Expertise: The true essence of nursing art'. *Advances in Nursing Science*, **17** (1), 15–24.

Hieghley, B. & Ferentz, T. (1988) 'Aesthetic inquiry' in Sarter, B. (ed.) *Paths to Knowledge*. New York: National League for Nursing Press. p. 11–144.

Johns, C. & Freshwater, D. (1998). *Transforming Nursing through Reflective Practice*. London: Blackwell Science.

Johnson, J.L. (1994) 'A dialectical examination of nursing art'. *Advances in Nursing Science*, **17** (1), 1–14.

Kazanis, B. (1992) *Personal Communication*. Tampa, FL: University of South Florida College of Education.

Kennick, W.E. (1979) *Art and Philosophy*. New York: St. Martin's Press.

Lange, S.P. (1990) 'Using the arts in clinical practice' in Leininger, M. & Watson, J. (eds). *The Caring Imperative in Education*. New York: National League for Nursing. p. 195–205.

Leininger, M.M. (1991) *Culture Care Diversity & Universality: A Theory of Nursing*. New York: National League for Nursing Press.

LeVasseur, J. (1999) 'Toward an understanding of art in nursing' *Advances in Nursing Science*, **21**: 4, 48–62.

Libby, D.B. (1992) 'Good morning', in *Nightingale Songs*, **2** (3), 4, P.O. Box 057563, West Palm Beach, FL. 33405.

Locsin, R. (1998) 'Aesthetic expression'. *International Journal for Human Caring*, **2** (1), 40–42.

Madayag, T.M. (1993) 'Isolation precautions' in *Nightingale Songs*, **2** (4), 1, P.O. Box 057563, West Palm Beach, FL. 33405.

Mayeroff, M. (1971) *On Caring*. New York: HarperCollins.

Moore, T. (1992) *Care of the Soul*. New York: HarperCollins.

Newman, M.A. (1994) *Health as Expanding Consciousness*. New York: National League for Nursing Press.

Oetting, P.C. (1991) 'Love is a small spoon' in *Nightingale Songs*, **1** (3), 2, P.O. Box 057653, West Palm Beach, FL. 33405.

Oiler, C. (1983) 'Nursing reality as reflected in nurse' poetry'. *Perspectives in Psychiatric Care*, **21** (3), 81–9.

Parker, M.E. (1992) 'Exploring the aesthetic meaning of presence in nursing practice' in Gaut, D.A. (ed.). *The Presence of Caring in Nursing*. New York: National League for Nursing Press. p. 25–37.

Parker, M.E. (1994a) 'Living nursing's values in nursing practice' in Gaut, D.A. & Boykin, A. (eds). *Caring as Healing: Renewal Through Hope*. New York: National League for Nursing Press. p. 48–65.

Parker, M.E. (1994b) 'The healing art of clay: A workshop for remembering wholeness' in Gaut, D.A. & Boykin, A. (eds). *Caring as Healing: Renewal Through Hope*. New York: National League for Nursing Press. p. 135–45.

Parker, M.E. (2001) *Nursing Theories and Nursing Practice*. Philadelphia: F.A. Davis, Co.

Parker, M.E. & Barry, C. (1999) 'Community practice guided by a nursing model'. *Nursing Science Quarterly*, **12** (2), 125–31.

Parker, M.E., Barry, C. & King, B. (2000) 'Use of inquiry method for assessment and evaluation in a school-based community nursing project'. *Family and Community Health*, **23** (2), 54–61.

Parker, M.E. & Schoenhofer, S. (1990) *Nightingale Songs*. P.O. Box 057563, West Palm Beach, FL. (www.fau.edu/divdept/nursing/ngsongs/nighting.htm).

Philosophy (1994) College of Nursing, Florida Atlantic University, Boca Raton, FL.

Progoff, I. (1971a) *The Star and the Cross: An Entrance Meditation*. New York: Dialogue House Library.

Progoff, I. (1971b) 'The center point within me' in *The Well and The Cathedral: An Entrance Meditation*. New York: Dialogue House Library. p. 59–86.

Ray, M.A. (2000). 'The theory of bureaucratic caring' in Parker, M. *Nursing Theories and Nursing Practice*. Philadelphia: F.A. Davis. p. 422–31.

Richards, M.C. (1962) *Centering in Pottery, Poetry and the Person*. Middletown, CT: Wesleyan University Press.

Roach, Sister M.S. (1987) *The Human Act of Caring*. Ottawa: Canadian Hospital Association.

Schoenhofer, S. (1989) 'Love, beauty, and truth: Fundamental nursing values'. *Nursing Education*, **28** (8), 392–384.

Schuster, E. (1998) 'Caring for Self: Working from the Inside Out'. Paper Presented at the International Association for Human Caring Research Conference, Philadelphia, June 1998.

Smith, M.J. (1992) 'Enhancing Aesthetic knowledge: A teaching strategy'. *Advances in Nursing Science*, **14** (3), 52–9.

Swanson, K.M. (1993) 'Nursing as informed caring for the well-being of others'. *Image: Journal of Nursing Scholarship*, **25**: 3, 352–7.

Tolstoy, L. (1930) *What is Art? And Essays on Art*. London: Oxford University Press.

Tomas, V. (1968) 'Creativity in art'. *The Philosophical Review*, **67**, 1–15.

Wagner, A.L. (2000) 'Connecting to nurse-self through reflective poetic story'. *International Journal for Human Caring*, **4** (2), 7–12.

Wainwright, P. (2000) 'Towards an aesthetics of nursing'. *Journal of Advanced Nursing*, **32** (3), 750–55.

Watson, J. (1999) *Postmodern nursing and beyond*. London: Churchill.

Watson, J. (2001). 'Theory of human caring' in Parker, M. *Nursing Theories and Nursing Practice*. Philadelphia: F.A. Davis, Co. pp. 344–60.

7 Nursing Students' Development of Caring Self Through Creative Reflective Practice

A. Lynne Wagner

The task of nursing education is to prepare competent caring nurses. Caring, more holistic than the narrowly focused technical competency of curing, is described as the essence of nursing, the paradigm for nursing practice (Saewye, 2000; Watson, 1988b). Recognized as a multidimensional concept that encompasses scientific, artful, personal, and moral components, caring denotes a therapeutic relationship between two or more people that is long-lasting in its healing effects (Bishop & Scudder, 1990; Carper, 1978; Watson, 1988a; 1999). Each caring encounter encompasses a reciprocal response between the persons involved that is often unpredictable and unique and therefore challenges the nurse to adaptively respond to each situation (Noddings, 1984; Schön, 1987).

Nursing involves interrelating personal self with professional self (Wagner, 2000). Most conceptual definitions of caring and lists of caring behaviors identify the use of self as a major component in establishing an adaptive therapeutic relationship. It is through the use of nurse-self that nursing science is artfully and therapeutically applied in each unique situation. The emphasis of knowing the personal or self, however, is not as firmly placed in nursing curricula as is knowing the empirical or nursing science (Bevis & Watson, 1989). Students need time to explore the concept of caring from a personal perspective and encouragement to develop adaptive caring practices that are artful and relational. This chapter explores the concept of self and the use of creative reflection as a means to increase nursing students' awareness of the impact of self in caring relationships.

The self in caring relationships

Rooted in humanistic and interpersonal theories, caring has been defined broadly as philosophical and theoretical constructs, and more definitively as specific behaviors. Implicitly threaded throughout definitions of caring is the need to develop a sense of self, a sense of knowing one's beliefs and values, intention to help, moral commitment to be present, ability to respond competently to another's need, and willingness to enter therapeutic relationships that encourage human connectedness.

One modern-day philosopher to explore the meaning and nature of caring is Milton Mayeroff in his work *On Caring*. Defining caring 'as helping other grow' (1971: 7), Mayeroff asserts that caring for another, a developmental process, gives meaning and order to one's own continuity of being. As a unique experience that honors personal separateness, caring nonetheless elicits a basic, common pattern of boundedness between persons through the purposeful being present for others in need. The reciprocity of caring resembles the flow of dancing together. As Mayeroff puts it:

> I experience the other as an extension of myself and also as independent and with the need to grow; I experience the other's development as bound up with my sense of well-being; and I feel needed by it for the growing. I respond affirmatively and with devotion to the other's need, guided by the direction of its growth. (1971: 11–12).

Mayeroff's (1971) eight major ingredients of caring include several references to the importance of knowing self in this partnership of caring. For example, the carer needs to adjust own behavior as the needs of others change (alternating rhythms), be self-confident in allowing another to find own way of growing (patience, trust), understand self and motives for helping (honesty), acknowledge own capabilities and limitations of helping based on past experiences and present situations (trust, humility), and nourish within oneself a sense of wonder for the present and a sense of future possibilities (hope, courage). Each characteristic helps the carer fine-tune the caring.

Another well-referenced contributor to the study of caring is Nel Noddings (1984), educator and ethicist. She also describes caring as a reciprocating, responsive relationship between two persons or parties, where there is an intention to care that is received and acknowledge by the cared-for. Caring is not fulfilled unless both dancers are involved (Noddings, 1984). Like Mayeroff (1971), Noddings states that 'caring involves stepping out of one's own personal frame of reference into the other's. When we care, we consider the other's point of view, his objective needs, and what he expects of us' (1981: 145). This subsumes that the carer needs to know one's own personal viewpoints and abilities, and needs to understand relational aspects of boundedness to others.

In addition, existential philosophers and the feminist theorists contribute to understanding the use of self in caring relationships. Key concepts in nursing caring models incorporate Heidegger's (1962) explorations of being-in-the-world, of being engaged in relationships, as well as Buber's (1953) relational distinction between the connecting I–Thou and distancing I–It perspectives. Rollo May posits that personal knowing emanates from participating in the world 'for to be in one's world means at the same time to be designing it' (1994: 123). Feminist theorists further expand the notion that caring emerges from a non-rational sense of nurturance (Noddings, 1984). Carol Gilligan (1982) differentiates the male objective, rational approach to relationships and the female nonlinear, nurturing approach that incorporates the more emotional subjective responsiveness of interpersonal relationships.

Likewise, nurses have molded definitions of caring with similar emphasis on self-awareness, use of therapeutic self, and relationship. Gaut (1983) identifies the use of self in caring encounters as an intentional act to care for another person that involves responsibility, awareness of and concern for the other person, and feelings of attachment. These characteristics are further summarized by Roach's (1992) five personal attributes of caring that demand insight of one's feelings, values, ability, and respect for others through compassion, competence, confidence, conscience, and commitment. In examining 35 definitions of caring, Morse et al. (1990) identify affect and interpersonal relationship among the five components the definitions share. Similarly, Benner & Wrubel (1989) espouse that caring involves knowing each patient's unique need to cope or grieve or heal, 'being with' a person in an engaged way and 'doing for' a person by meeting mutually planned goals (1989: 5). One can only know or be with another in this relational way through self-understanding and self-disclosure (Jourard, 1964).

Watson's (1988a; 1988b) definition of caring includes deeper emphasis on discovery of self and intersubjective meaning of nurse–patient relationships amidst health–illness situations. She describes caring actions as interactive and embedded in a metaphysical, transpersonal relationship. These actions, based on knowledge and respect of self and other, are driven by a moral intention to preserve human dignity. The professional work of caring 'requires personal, social, moral and spiritual engagement' (Watson, 1988b: 29). The nurse's intent is to accurately recognize the subjective significance of illness for another, to feel a mutuality with the person, and to know one's self, identifying one's ability or inability to respond. Transpersonal caring represents a meeting of two spirits, a human, often spiritual encounter that is contextual, temporal, but lasting in its imprint and ability to move each person toward a higher sense of self and harmony. According to Watson (1999), the caring moment occurs when the carer and the cared for enter each other's phenomenal space, that in turn creates a new space and opportunity for being with each other. Nursing as a human science of care challenges one to understand not only what nurses do, but more importantly, what it means to be a caring nurse, what it means to bring oneself to nursing to effect a transformative relationship of healing (Watson, 1999).

Ways of knowing caring self

Knowledge building and ways of knowing caring self are complex personal and collective processes embedded in one's practice of caring for others. Carper (1978) proposed four interrelated fundamental patterns of knowing in nursing that incorporate the empirics or science of nursing (factual knowledge), the esthetics or art of nursing (experiential ways of doing), personal knowledge or knowledge of self, and ethical knowledge or the moral component. These four components of caring give nursing a particular perspective and significance as a profession, with an emphasis on the development of therapeutic nurse self.

Traditionally, the emphasis of nursing education has focused heavily on the first component, the science of nursing, a reflection of the medical model: 'rationalizing and compartmentalizing the care of patients' (Tanner, 1988). This suggests nursing education has neglected to fully prepare nurses in developing their experiential art of caring, the power of personal knowledge and mastery, and the moral valuing that is necessary when caring for human life (Noddings, 1984; Watson, 1988b, 1999). Since the 1970s, nursing leaders have amassed a voice to challenge the narrow focus and reclaim the holistic primacy of competent caring in nursing. Silva et al. (1995) applaud Carper's seminal work on the fundamental patterns of knowing. However, the authors discuss the philosophical shift in nursing from epistemology to ontology, turning the question of 'How do I come to know nursing?' to 'How do I find meaning in what I know?', 'What does it mean to care?' Roach (1991: 8) asks in a similar ontological manner: 'What is the "being" of caring?'

The knowing of self, or personal knowing, so intricately tied into becoming nurse, is enmeshed in multiple and changing realities of relationships (Schön, 1987). The Human Nursing Theory (Paterson and Zderad, 1976) describes personal knowing on three levels: objective (outside-in perspective, observed, non-personal); subjective (inside out perspective, self-awareness); and intersubjective (relational perspective, exchanging, responsive). Recognizing that each level fosters insight, it is the intersubjective process that reveals the fullest possibility for caring (Wagner, 2000; Watson, 1999). Bishop and Scudder (1990) acknowledge that personal knowing in nursing includes understanding self in relationship with patients and being openly respectful and responsive to the uniqueness of each relationship. Holden (1996) further supports this view, arguing that subjective, affective knowledge blends with the practical, cultural and perceptual levels of nursing knowledge to allow for a more holistic approach to nursing practice.

Rollo May, who explores the evolving 'consciousness of self', posits that for humans to 'love our neighbor, to have ethical sensitivity, to see truth, to create beauty, to devote ourselves to ideals' (1973: 86), one must step beyond merely seeing the other (objective) and empathize with others (intersubjective). Likewise, Benner and Wrubel (1989) acknowledge that the art of empathy is an important ingredient of caring and allows the nurse to relate to a person's struggles in connecting human ways. Furthermore, May states that the 'self is always born in a social context' of interpersonal relationships (1973: 88). He contends, however, that selfhood evolves from a uniquely personal journey and can be destroyed by social conformity. As such, the development of nurse-self in relation to each nursing encounter needs to be honored as unique and changing.

Thus knowing nurse-self is a process that occurs within the context of multiple ways of knowing relational self. How one comes to know self in this context is not clear. It is argued that reflection on clinical practice is one valuable way to integrate the cognitive, affective, and cultural components of caring (Benner, 1984; Bishop & Scudder, 1990; Johns, 1994a; 1998a; Leininger, 1988; Schön, 1987). Metcalfe (1990) explores five dimensions of the learning process in clinical practice. Two specific dimensions focus on knowledge of self and relationship through reflection. *Focused deliberation* refers to increased cognitive and caring awareness that occurs with self-reflection and group discussion on nursing experiences. A second dimension, *insight dissemination,* occurs when information and skills are applied to new situations and the student or nurse sees that one nurse–patient relationship, although a unique experience, can inform the next relationship. Metcalfe describes this as an aesthetic level of '*body and mind* coming together in a way of knowing' (1990: 151).

Dewey (1933; 1934) explores how a person thinks and uses creative reflection to examine thoughts, experiences and feelings in search for meaning of an experience. Likewise, acknowledging that knowing self has important impact on self-concept and self-image and ultimately on one's relationship with the world, psychologists have pursued self-reflection as an important process of becoming, of knowing self and the impact of self on personal and social encounters (Allport, 1955; James, 1929). Jourard claims that self-disclosure is important to growth of self. Specifically referring to nursing, he states:

> Knowing patients calls for inquiry … general nursing calls for the ability to see that which is common to all mankind in oneself and in the other person. This means that to know all mankind one begins by looking within oneself. (1964: 140)

Belenky et al. (1986) add still another dimension to understanding how reflection aids a nurse in knowing caring-self. In their study of women's ways of knowing, they describe five patterns of increasing self-awareness as one moves from passive to active knowing. Constructed knowledge is the highest level gained through integrating and contextually applying subjective and procedural knowledge. Such growth toward constructing a more holistic knowledge about one's caring practice can be fostered through reflection and dialogue.

Although reflection-in-action has been identified as an important step in becoming an expert nurse (Benner, 1984; Schön, 1983; 1987), reflection-on-action is foundational to nursing education to help students construct their rational and affective knowledge. Students need a supportive environment to reflect on their practice retrospectively and to process newly gained understanding with faculty and peers. Both the personal reflecting and the shared dialogue enriches self-awareness and enlarges the perspective of therapeutic self amidst the changing reality of patient care and the possibilities for future practice.

Johns (1994a; 1998b), who works with nurses in individual and group guided-reflection sessions, developed a Structured Reflection Model. He describes reflective practice as a critical thinking process that 'involves the practitioner paying attention to significant aspects of experience in order to make sense of it within the context of their intention' (1994a: 7). This requires the practitioner to be honest and confrontational with self to understand contradictions of what is practiced and what is desirable. Based on the basic assumptions that reflection is a process of revealing new insights, that nurses are capable of being reflective and creative, and that reflection-on-actions guides future caring practice, Johns (1994b) purports that personal or group reflection fosters intrapersonal knowing of self; interpersonal knowing of therapeutic self in context with the patient, and intra/interpersonal knowing therapeutic self in partnership with others.

The reflective process occurs on different levels. Freshwater (2001), Gibbs (1988) and Goodman (1984) identify three such levels. The first is a descriptive level that describes the situation, techniques, skills, relationships and feelings. The second level is an evaluative phase that challenges one to examine relationships between self and practice and contradictions between the espoused theories learned in class and the theories-in-use utilized in clinical practice (Argyris & Schön, 1974). A more expansive third level examines ethical and political influences on care that extend beyond the actual experience (Goodman, 1984), as well as proposes needed changes (Freshwater, 2001; Gibbs, 1988). These levels, often overlapping in a reflective exercise, directs the nurse to reflect on practice in order to increase self-awareness of strengths and limitations, to integrate theory and practice, and to foster different perspectives and creative alternative approaches to nursing practice.

Powell (1989) posits that students need an awareness of experience and the ability to describe difficult but key caring moments. Powell finds in her study of eight nurses and their use of reflection during daily practice that learning opportunities existing in everyday work situations are not always recognized nor acknowledged as growing experiences. She implores nursing educators to help students examine their practice, asking the *why* of nursing care, as well as the *how* and *what*. Dewey (1938) described the attitudes needed for reflection as open mindedness, responsibility to examine ideas beyond the context, and wholeheartedness of commitment.

Reflective opportunities in nursing education

It is recognized that a caring self can be fostered through education, role modeling, dialogue and practice (Green-Hernandez, 1991; Leininger, 1988; 1995; Metcalfe, 1990; Noddings, 1986). Leininger's (1981; 1985; 1991) work toward a culture-care theory adds to the understanding that caring is both an innate and learned human behavior. Leininger's (1981) professional *care* and *professional nurse caring* levels expand the innate sense of *generic caring* through knowledge-building and clinical practice. Likewise, Benner's (1984) work on growth from novice to expert nurse demonstrates that nurses learn to care through both education and practice over time.

Thus curriculum design is an important aspect of teaching caring. The model of diagnostic reasoning and scientific problem solving, that has been traditionally used to teach the nursing process, does not encourage humanistic inquiry (Watson, 1988a), holistic judgments (Benner, 1984; Holden, 1996) or pattern recognition of culture care (Leininger, 1991; Tanner 1988). Watson (1988a) challenges nursing education to create a 'new professional nurse' who understands the 'moral context of health and human caring in nursing' (1988a: 424). Among suggestions for nursing curricula changes, both Watson (1999) and Young-Mason (1988; 1995) propose the need to acknowledge the arts and humanities as essential elements for caring professionals. Watson (1994; 1999) further proposes the fostering of faculty and student creativity and co-authorship in the study of caring-healing behaviors. The implication of this call for change is the need to a develop a more creative, collaborative and relational pedagogy in nursing, helping students to construct and integrate knowledge of self, values and art with the science.

Bevis (1989) suggests that active involvement in such activities as discovery learning, modeling and heuristics can heighten a student's learning, connecting nursing theory to practice, science to art, and self to other. Discovery learning is guided activities that challenge students to synthesize information and generate alternative solutions, opening the process to aesthetic and personal knowing. Modeling incorporates the ideas of learning from teacher and fellow students through example and of cooperative inquiry (Heron, 1981a; 1981b). Heuristic activities engage the student to explore an idea, goal, or problem. Such activities include the use of reflective journaling and narrative to increase students' self-awareness of the meaning and impact of their caring (Beckerman, 1994; Freshwater, 1998a; 1998b; Parker, 1992; Vaught-Alexander, 1994; Wagner, 1998).

Journaling and written or verbal narratives are well-accepted reflective tools in nursing education (Diekelmann 1993; Freshwater, 1998b; Noddings, 1992). In reviewing the literature, Nehls (1995) summarizes that educational narrative approaches include anecdotes, critical incidents in clinical practice, paradigm cases and journals. Higgins (1996) reports success in awakening nursing student's caring values by inviting them to tell their stories of caring as they dealt with uncomfortable nursing situations. Baker (1996) and Saylor (1990) also use reflective journaling of clinical experiences to expand the narrow tendency of students to report only on their tasks. Likewise, Gunby (1994) finds that insight into nursing students' experiences in caring for ill and suffering patients is gained via their narratives of their lived experiences. Parker (1990) reminds educators that subjective narratives or stories are recognized as only representative of the experience perceived at the time of the telling. Stories are not time-bound. They have a life of their own and often change in the process of telling (Vezeau, 1993). Lanzara (1991) calls this phenomenon 'shifting stories'. Their truth comes by virtue of what is important enough to remember (Sandelowski, 1996; Vezeau, 1994). In the end, perception of the event is what affects one's behavior.

Reflection on literature, poetry and the arts is documented as a powerful vehicle to increase self-awareness and connectedness to other human beings. As reflective expressions, art and poetry capture the artist's personal experiences in representative images (Dewey, 1934; Wagner, 2000). 'Art-making' is a process, a journey for both artist and viewer. As such, 'art can be appreciated for its dynamic portrayal of the changing human condition that has been stilled only by its own framing' (Wagner, 2000: 9). Artistic expression speaks a truth that invites others to explore and expand the artist's story by adding their own and thereby raising human consciousness to new levels of wholeness (Chinn, 1994).

The study of art and the humanities bridges personal and aesthetic knowing, for in interpreting art, people find a part of themselves, a part of their story, in the image the artist puts before them. Bartol (1986), Bergman and Krant (1977), Young-Mason (1995), and Darbyshire (1994) explore the use of the humanities in nursing education as a means to gain insight into and a sensitivity for human behavior and emotions surrounding health and illness, birthing and dying, growth and loss. Students evaluate these learning experiences as positive and enjoyable and as informative and illustrative of the complexity of human experience (Cassidy, 1996; Darbyshire, 1994).

Both Darbyshire (1994; 1995) and Young-Mason (1995) further acknowledge that the power of recognizing human conditions in literary works or art and of empathizing with the characters comes not only from relating to personal nursing experiences but, more importantly, from dialogue with others about the insights. Creating the course *Understanding Caring Through Arts and the Humanities,* Darbyshire (1994) uses literary texts, paintings and photography to stimulate nursing students' artistic and aesthetic sense of being human, of being nurse, patient, ill, disabled. This sense of self as human is internalized through reflective comparisons with the students' own nursing world and through a dialogical approach, aimed not at consensus, but at openness to the multiplicity of interpretations. Darbyshire (1995), like Bevis, emphasizes the importance of the teacher as an active participant in creating the 'conditions and possibilities whereby nursing humanities can work' (1989: 214).

Another strategy for aesthetic exploration in nursing education is encouraging students to interpret their caring encounters through personal creative expression. The experience of creating images through poetry and art-making from the inside-out, rather than viewing another artist's work from the outside-in, creates a different avenue for self-awareness and personal knowing. In art therapy, creating art has proved to be a powerful healing vehicle for communicating suppressed feelings and thoughts that are often too deep and painful to be expressed in words (Freshwater, 1999; Lynn, 1995; Samuels, 1995; Sheppard, 1994). The creation of art in many forms of drawing, painting, photography, clay, music, dance, poetry and story has been used in intervention programs with addicts (Feen-Calligan, 1995), cancer patients (Predeger, 1996; Ziesler, 1993), Alzheimer patients (Sterritt & Pokorny, 1994), children and adults experiencing grief (Bertman, 1991; Davis, 1989; Harr & Thistlethwaite, 1990), professionals counseling the bereaved (Zamierowski & Gordon, 1995) and victims of child abuse (Cumbie & Rutherford, 1994; Estep, 1995). Art as therapy is based on the continual demonstration that people can move expressions of the unconscious psyche to the surface through creative process (McNiff, 1992). The creating of art is a reflective process, which McNiff calls 'dialoguing with images … a method for expanding the ego's singular vision' (1992: 2).

Personal knowing through creative expression is further expanded when the journey of discovery is shared in a dialogic group experience (Cumbie & Rutherford, 1994; Darbyshire, 1994; 1995; McNiff, 1992; Young-Mason, 1995). Predeger (1996), in her work with survivors of breast cancer, finds that creating art in a group helped these woman gain control in their lives, illuminated a changing life perspective, moved them to be proactive rather than reactive to their illness, and created a relational connectedness with others in a safe setting for deep exploration of their feelings. Through photography, watercolor, collage, poetry and word images, these women dialogued, reflected and discovered new meaning to their lives and to their relations with others.

Thus the creation of art itself is therapeutic and educative in its centering and expanding capacities. However, personal reflection on the process and collective dialogue with others appear to be important additional steps in gaining an increased understanding of self in the world. Reflection on the ordinary can be as revealing as exploring the extraordinary. Nurses who have allowed the nurse and the artist in them to meet, have new reflective opportunities to expand their worldview.

Nurse as artist

Nurse-artists provide insight into the role of the arts in nursing education through the aesthetic sense they bring to nursing. In fact, Parker (1992) claims that all nurses are artists. Many nurse-artists discover the power and impact of creative expression by using it reflectively during personal struggle in practice (Lane, 1994). Breunig (1994) relates how painting allows her to know herself and her nursing practice. Painting helps her center; to be attentive; gives her perspective of the aesthetic human world amid the technical wizardry. It enables her to coexist with anxiety and pain, giving each their respectful space on her empty canvas without crowding out the other important aspects of her life. In essence, through her painting she finds her authentic self and the strength to practice her caring.

In my own work as a nurse-poet I attempt to see patterns and metaphors in women's stories about their journey with breast cancer (Wagner, 1995) and in nurses' stories about caring for dying patients (Wagner, 1999). I create a cyclic poetic dialogue that encompasses listening to a story, poetically reflecting on the story, and inviting the storyteller to reflect on the poetry. This circular dialogue creates space and openness for a deeper understanding of the story, enlarging the story's meaning as it evolves and creating new possibilities for nurse–patient relationships.

Nurse-artist Lane (1994) used her art background to establish an Artist in Residence Program in a bone-marrow transplant unit, promoting healing through the creative arts. Picard (2000a) a nurse-dancer, recognizes that movement is 'a lived body experience' (1994: 148) and through movement a person contracts and expands space, experiencing vulnerability or exposure in the relative space with others. Bringing this understanding to her nursing practice, Picard has a heightened appreciation of patients' body-experience during illness. Parker's (1994) experience with clay helps her to understand centering and transpersonal relationships. A hermeneutic inquiry of five nurse-artists (Parker, 1992) explores the impact of creating art on nursing practice. Through reflective journaling, these nurse-artists report on the blending of boundaries with the art teaching about balance and the nursing teaching about sensitivity, openness to ideas, and being present. Both nursing and art are perceived as holistically connected to healing. The power of artistic expression is its ability to tap greater depth of details, emotions and meaning attached to experiences than casual description reveals. Patients who use art as therapy, students who use art as learning about themselves and their world, and nurse-artists who use art to understand their practice and communicate with others, all experience this power of aesthetic personal knowing (Skillman-Hull, 1994).

Knowing self at greater depths is exemplified through the following case study of one student's experience reflecting on practice through creating and sharing of story, poetry and art. This case is part of a larger multi-case qualitative research study (Wagner, 1998) that explored creative expression as a reflective pedagogical approach in a RN to BSN nursing program. The students were enrolled in a 14-week Holistic Nursing course that met biweekly. An assignment for each class over the semester was to write a story about a caring (or uncaring) encounter with a patient, translate that story into art or poetry (as assigned by the teacher), and share both the story and creative expression in class. As the facilitator of the course I explained that creative expression for these exercises has no rules nor requires any special artistic ability. I also stressed that the important part of the exercise is the process of creating, not the product (poem or artwork). Data collected include transcribed field notes from each class meeting, three personal interviews with each participant over the semester, the students' stories and creative expressions, and the reflective journals the students kept during the experience. The representative example presented below, demonstrates students' growing awareness of self as nurse and as co-partner in therapeutic nurse–patient relationships.

A case study

Tori (pseudonym) is a 23-year-old, single, diploma-prepared nurse with two and half years of nursing experience in an acute care rehabilitation setting. She is working full-time while she attends a baccalaureate nursing program part-time. She cared for people 'as she would want to be cared for'. Also evident in her stories and dialogue with classmates was a strong sense of family values. She admitted she felt burned-out after only two years in nursing due to the increased workload and stresses in nursing. She had returned to school to try to 'refuel' herself. Three representative examples of Tori's process are presented.

Story and poetry

For one of her poetry-writing assignments, Tori chose a story that represents a constant pet peeve. Initially giving a 'nurse's report' of the patient's condition as background, Tori then centers her story on her response to an 'uncaring' nursing situation between a patient and a nursing assistant.

It was about 45 minutes prior to the end of the shift. As the nursing assistant was beginning to turn the patient, who was nonverbal, she stated very loudly and in a tone which echoed that of disgust, 'Oh, great, she's dirty again.' Tori expressed her own anger and sadness at this inhuman treatment and then empathized with the patient, giving the story voice.

I quickly snapped: 'She can't help it. When you're her age and in her condition, do you want your nursing assistant to treat you like that?' At that moment, I was very angry and sad. Although the patient was nonverbal, she could still comprehend what was going on around her. I thought, 'What must she be feeling at this time – sadness, anger, embarrassment?' I turned to the patient and said, 'Don't worry, we'll clean you up so you'll be more comfortable.'

The reflective poem was a deeper, more powerful statement than found in the story itself of Tori's holistic, caring philosophy that honors the personhood and respect of the patient and reveals her emotions stirred by the uncaring. Thoughtfully crafted through voice and image, the untitled poem transcends the particular incident in the story to symbolize the universal human plight of the aging person who needs care. The perspective of the poem moved from the empathetic voice and questions of the young nurse, to the projections of an aging patient who has journeyed through life, to the universal nurse:

I am young, just 23, but at times I THINK as if I were old.
I think of the days ahead and of those that will be my last.
How will they be? I think …

I imagine, MY GREATEST FEAR,
to be old, alone, lying in bed with no loved ones within reach,
at the mercy of people who see me as those who saw her:
    as a bother,
    as an inconvenience,
at the mercy of people who talk ABOUT ME BUT NOT TO ME,
at the mercy of those who look AT ME BUT DO NOT SEE ME.

TO THOSE PEOPLE, I WANT TO SCREAM:
I was once as young as you – vibrant and independent.
You see a frail old woman,
who no longer speaks, no longer self feeds,
who no longer bathes or dresses herself.
You do not see me.
I am an educated scholar who influenced young minds.
I am a wife, a mother, a friend, a pianist.
Over the years MY BODY HAS FAILED ME, NOT MY MIND.
When you speak to me,
when you groan and sigh because it takes longer
and longer each day to feed me,
and when you complain because I am incontinent …

JUST REMEMBER,
    THERE IS MORE TO ME THAN YOU CHOOSE TO SEE.
    Believe me, I never thought I would one day be like this.
When you look at me, THINK …
    YOU COULD BE LOOKING AT YOURSELF IN 50 YEARS!

The poem's power and depth of feelings come from Tori's value system that was bruised by the particular incident, but did not come to full realization until she wrote the poem. The poem allowed Tori to be reflective of what it is like to be a patient. Her voice welled up from a conscious level of again being there with the patient. She explains the process of poetry-making as lengthy and somewhat difficult, but she admitted it became easier. In fact, in testimony to the power of image and feeling that the poetry-making elicited, she admitted at the last interview that she wrote the poetry before the story. The poem served as an outline for crafting the story.

Tori stated that the poetry 'was a group of words describing her intense emotions or feelings' that she could not express in the story. There was a freedom for 'creative expressive outlet' that transcended the normal rules of narrative:

> The story is sitting there … with the poem you have more freedom to express your deep thoughts and feelings by the way you accentuate words … There is much more [emotion] in writing the poetry as opposed to the whole narrative. If you just write one word, it has that much more power than writing the whole story, with sentences and correct grammar.

The reflective process of the poetry-making was revealing and healing to this participant. The personal meaning of the process was in the release of her emotions and an increased self-awareness of their existence and depth:

> The poetry enabled me to let go of feelings that I've had, like anger … I've been able to write it and put it aside … I still think of it, but I wasn't as angry because I was able to get it out on paper and express myself and handle it in a different way … I just released it, you know, got it away from me … let go of it. I could then move on. I think as nurses we are taught not to listen to our emotions.

Furthermore, there was meaning in the process on a professional level, with an increased awareness of her accumulative experiences and their impact on her caring practice.

> Thinking about the story and especially writing the poem made me think about my role in caring and how I can get others to understand about patients like this. I don't usually think about things like this so deeply … Writing the poem forced me to look inside my story and see how I handled myself. The poem helped me relieve the stress in that situation and gave me direction in what to do next time.

Story and art

Tori's art projects centered on the creation of art from her stories of two caring moments that represented to her 'just routine days with no big deal'. Although she recognized the inherent caring in her actions, through processing these stories on different levels of reflection she realized a new perspective of her caring, a transpersonal relationship with her patients. The process was complex.

Tori chose to write about a patient who had been a difficult challenge for her. She introduced the patient as difficult and described her own frustrations as a nurse. Having set the scene of the story, Tori then related a change in their relationship, precipitated by Tori's reaching out to this patient, without her understanding the significance of her action.

One day, things changed. I don't know what happened, but we began a reciprocal relationship. She actually began to grin and stick her tongue out at me, which was a positive response. We began to do activities that increase her feeling of wellbeing. I began to paint her nails, put lipstick on her and bring her in earrings to wear. Her tears have decreased and she uses less pain medication. Granted some days are better than others, but overall we have now begun a new relationship with better understanding of each other. We now communicate and talk not only about her medical condition, but also about the weather, news, visits with her brother.

After reading her story in class, discussion prompted Tori to divulge more details about the incident. Through continued dialogic processing, Tori became aware of the significance of her actions.

The social worker one day noticed that the patient was eyeing my nail polish and made a comment, 'Do you like having nail polish?' So the next day, I got an idea to bring in my nail polish and did her nails. That was the moment things changed.

The art translation of this story, a type of collage, was not a difficult activity for Tori, but required a thoughtful process to depict the key elements and mood in the story.

I didn't want to make everything real bright because the situation isn't all that bright yet, you know. The art piece symbolizes a 'sunshine face', representing her new smiles, but still gray days in her rays. Earrings are the eyes and a bottle of nail polish and tube of lipstick are 'central to her face'. A pain pill, 'which she needs less of now', is off to the side of her cheek, almost as a blemish. The card and comb represent caring.

In processing this story, Tori gained new meaning in what she began to realize was an unroutine nursing action. Tori discovered a deeper sense of relationships in her nursing through translating the story into art and then sharing the story and art in class.

The art with all the symbolism really made me think that much more about the relationship. Even after I had written the story, I remember that I didn't know exactly what had occurred. I was just reporting facts. In doing my poster, I realized there was a turning point [in our relationship]. But I didn't know why it had happened; I just knew that it occurred. Then by sharing my story and art in class with everybody giving feedback, I understood that I had crossed over into her life by bringing in the nail polish and the lipstick. I connected with her.

Tori's second story-to-art project further illustrated this new appreciation of how a nurse's seemingly insignificant actions are often meaningful caring moments. The experience happened almost a year before, but was remembered for the difference Tori made in her patient's life. Caring on Christmas Day for a newly-admitted man who was recovering from severe injuries, Tori very briefly introduced the patient by medical diagnoses. She then focused on the patient's and his wife's high anxiety, their close relationship, and their needs:

That afternoon his wife came in to see him. Around 2 p.m. he was going to take a nap. He was in a two-bed room with the second bed unoccupied. His wife, looking very tired and worn, asked me if she could lie down for a few minutes in the unoccupied bed. I told her she could and returned a few minutes later and covered her over with a blanket.

> I closed the door and exited the room. During my last set of rounds, I peeked in the room and found both of them sleeping soundly. I didn't care if I got into trouble. She needed that bed.

Tori explained to the class that she felt her gesture at the time was nothing special. The patient, however, felt that her action was a special reaching out that connected her to their lives. Much to Tori's surprise, the patient stayed in touch with her after discharge.

> The next day the patient commented how impressed he was that I thought enough about him and his wife to give her a blanket. He commented on it several times that day. It caught me off guard; something that was so simple made such an impression on him.

This realization of the importance of her actions came through her creative expression.

> Sometimes I think I look at caring as more of a grander scheme of things, like saving someone's life. But of course that's not always necessary. I now realize with all this reflection that what you do in ten minutes with that person can be the difference for them and they can really feel well cared for … that caring moment can be the small things like, bringing the blanket to the person. To me that was nothing … just doing my job, to them it was a big deal … I know as a nurse what I wanted to accomplish … But I don't think I knew before this class the extent of what I was really doing in my nursing practice and how I was affecting people's lives and if I was … So through the poetry and art I looked at myself and knew I've had an impact on somebody's life to make it a little better for them.

After reading the story to the class, Tori introduced her drawing of the man and his wife in the side-by-side beds with snow falling outside the window and a symbolic Christmas tree on the windowsill. Unlike the poetry-making, writing the story first was of particular importance to hold the images in mind. She sifted through the story's detail to find the essence of the experience.

> For this assignment I needed the story in front of me as an outline … I remember in my head what my images are, but the art is harder to make images real-looking, the complete image. With poetry it is easier to say those images in words. For instance, how do you draw calmness? So I sifted through the story and just thought, What's going on here? What is the essence in this story? What's the right image? Then I drew that.

Despite her belief that she had no art ability and the frustration of creating the drawing (product), Tori very positively identified that the reflective process fostered of spending more time with the images helped her see the details of the experience better.

> The process was somewhat frustrating … I went through a couple of drafts trying to sketch things and then trying to get more detail-oriented and improve it that way. The time I spent laboring over it [the drawing] made me think more about the experience itself … When I started to create the drawing is when I realized that my everyday nursing really was a big deal to them.

While the poetry offered Tori an outlet for feelings and voice, the art-making provided a vehicle for choosing to display the essence of the story in a symbolic way. The process of sharing the art in class was different than the poetry sharing.

We spend more class time analyzing the art than the poetry. I think it has to do with the visual. When people see things, they gain more understanding; have more insight than if they just hear it [like the poetry] ... We're trying to find meaning in it for ourselves.

Sharing

Sharing the stories and artwork in class promoted yet a different level of collective reflection that enhanced personal knowing of caring-self. Sharing at this level of collective consciousness allowed for further personal reflection that had begun with the creating of the story and art, with the students going beyond questions of 'What is happening here?' to now asking such questions as 'Why did this happen?' or 'What could I have done better?'

Sharing also provided support and affirmation of each other's caring and nursing practice, as well as perspective of the nursing culture itself. One aspect of the supportive function that Tori described was the therapeutic release of emotions that the poetry and art sharing allowed.

The sharing is really good because I think in nursing you sometimes don't feel important. It's very stressful. You need people with whom you can share experiences. My family is supportive, but they just don't get it ... Before I started taking this class, I was actually thinking of moving out of nursing. I was feeling burned-out after two years. You're giving to everybody all day with no one to talk to – no release ... The creative stuff really brought out the emotions and feelings that nurses don't usually talk about ... I gain a lot by sharing the story and art and listening to people's reactions to it ... We helped each other. It has given me new hope that there are nurses out there who really do care and who are going through the same thing I am ... I don't feel as alone or that it is never going to get better.

Tori felt that the personal work at home creating the story and translating it into art were necessary precedents to presenting in class and allowing this next level of reflection. At the group reflection level, she enlarged her understanding of specific nursing experiences to encompass her larger nursing practice.

Discussion

Tori's experience is one example of reflection on practice through creative expression that helped her explore her therapeutic caring-self and the impact of her nurse-self in nurse–patient relationships. Her descriptions about the process support extant theories and experiential accountings of reflective practice. The case study also teaches more about the meaning of caring and the power reflection has to bring one's caring-self to full consciousness in practice.

Without a doubt, Tori is a caring nurse. She demonstrates respect, compassion and confidence in her unroutine actions, despite possible criticism from her co-workers, and a moral conscience in her motivations to help others (Mayeroff, 1971; Roach, 1992). She redesigned her behavior (nail polish and blanket stories) to meet the needs of her patients and their families (May, 1994). In each case, through non-rational nurturance (Gilligan, 1982), Tori's caring transcended her

Table 7.1   *Typology of reflective levels used to explore caring-self in*
nursing practice

Level of reflection	Reflective activity	Process	Outcome
Cognitive	Descriptive story-writing and telling of nursing experiences.	Rational process; recall of experiences; asks, 'What happened?'; remembering details; relives experience.	Organization of details; identifies self and others; experience available for deeper reflection.
Affective	Creative expression of experiences through poetry and art.	Non-rational analytic process; forced to go inside the story; confronts feelings and relationships; asks, 'What is going on here?', 'What is important?'; sifts through the detail of story to find 'essence' of experience.	Deeper relational meaning becomes known to self; connecting to patient; healing emotions; therapeutic.
Collective	Sharing stories; dialogue.	Allows self to be heard; Listens to others' stories; forms collective story; asks, 'Why did you do it that way?'; discovery of alternative ways of doing.	Therapeutic; support; revealing to others; connecting, circular; reaffirming.

technical competence when she stepped out of her personal frame and into the patient's or family member's phenomenal field (Watson, 1988b; 1999). However, what is significant is that she did not fully recognize her caring-self and her impact on her relationships. In her burned-out state, she had lost sight of who she was as caring-nurse, the importance of what she was doing, and hope for nursing as a profession. The reflective process that occurred on several levels helped her to find renewed meaning in caring-self and in nursing through an enlarged perspective on her caring.

Levels of reflection

Through story, creative expression and sharing, Tori reflected on three levels that are described as cognitive, affective and collective (Wagner, 1998). On each level, the reflective activity prompted a study of self or *selfology* through identified processes and outcomes. Each level provided increased understanding of therapeutic caring-self. This typology of the reflective levels is summarized in Table 7.1.

Reflecting through descriptive choosing and writing stories is a cognitive exercise of recall and reporting, which Banks-Wallace (1998) identifies as contextual grounding. This reflective step required remembering experiences, some of which were deeply buried in her subconscious, and resulted in organizing her accounts of the experience in a factual, orderly fashion.

I don't think about my experiences much. I just keep going. When I did try [to think], the experiences would kind of swim around in my head ... They were fragmented. But by doing the stories I have something in front of me that is organized and then I'm able to think about things more and analyze things more and then take all that information back in and that has increased my self-awareness.

Reconstructing her experience required Tori to travel from her outward stance inward, asking 'What is happening here?' It brought the unexplored details of an experience out of storage into the foreground and made them available for further reflecting on (Johns, 1994a; 1996). This cognitive level of reflection mirrors what Goodman (1984) referred to as descriptive and Habermas (1977) described as technical. According to Brookfield (1990), reflections that just report without attention to meaning are cognitive activities that provide factual, noncritical details or abstractions. Further reflection is needed to uncover meaning. The descriptive, noncritical framing of the story was an important preparatory step for the deeper reflective process that was to follow in Tori's use of artistic expression. By bringing the details to the surface again, the initial descriptive story, whether written or not, provided a more available database for the continuing process of reflection on the experience through poetry and art.

Creative reflection evoked the second level of affective insight that allowed deeper reflection; a vehicle to communicate newly surfaced feelings, a cathartic healing outlet. Tori described the deeper level of reflection that emerged from her search for the right words for the poems and the right images for the drawings. Her poetic reflections sprung from the heart, eliciting emotions of the experiences that had only been uncomfortably felt, but never expressed (Atkins & Murphy, 1993). She felt feelings could be explored, named and communicated through poetic use of words and grammatical structure. Feelings and questions of life's worth were honored and therapeutically released in the participant's poem of anger; of life's uncertainty, pain and suffering; of caring and uncaring touch. As such, without ever being poet before, her 'poetic heart' that the poet Tennyson (cited in Moyers, 1995: xvii) identified, spoke more deeply than did her cognitive mind through story. Fox finds poem-making a way to 'think by feeling' (1997: 33), thus giving voice to head through heart. David Whyte (1994) uses story through poetry to 'arouse the heart', to nourish the inner creative force that expresses our humanness in the often orderly, technical work world. The nurse-student observed that poetry, unencumbered by all the detail stuff in the story, allowed her creative poetic sense to reach what Whyte calls 'the underground forces' that shape daily life (1994: 5). In the same vein, Sandelowski found that artists eliminate 'trivial, transient elements' of an experience to illuminate the essence of life (1996: 113).

On the other hand, art-making, less emotional than the poetry, elicited a clearer vision of relationship than the story did. Tori felt her lack of artistic talent prevented her from expressing powerful emotions that are more easily conveyed through words. The art, however, forced Tori inside the story to capture the essence of the story. Tori's blanket story on Christmas Day stilled the motion of the story, portraying a mental photograph of one scene that represented the essence of the whole. She created image from insight (Miles, 1985) and dialogued with images (McNiff, 1992) in both artworks. The art made the image visible. Dulles claims that 'symbol introduces us to realms of awareness not normally accessible to discursive thought' and can foster insights from 'deeper aspects of reality' (1985: 137).

This process of going back inside the story, reliving the experience, visualizing herself in the situation again, seeing the experience anew, is akin to what Bevis (1989) calls 'discovery learning' and Goodman (1984) describes as the second level of examining the relationship between self and practice. The process opened a new vista for Tori in which to view more microscopically not only what was going on, but also how she was feeling, how the patient was feeling. It was personal, inside work. Her thinking expanded from describing 'What was happening?' to exploring 'What is important here?', 'What is the essence of this story?' The resulting poems and artwork, in turn, became outward expressions of the inside perspective, making visible what was invisible in the initial descriptive story. While the emotive poetry made the nurse's human side visible, the art made the patient as person visible.

Lastly, sharing fostered a third level of collective reflection. Sharing personal reflective artwork opened a deeper level of conversation than just reading the descriptive written story. Mezirow (1991) and Freshwater (2001; 1998b) refer to this as transformative emancipatory learning. As Tori indicated, listening and dialogue fostered a connecting with each other in that common space each knew as nursing where they found meaning (Isaacs, 1994). Through dialogue, students gained affirmation of who they were and what they did as nurses, support of their nursing, and a sisterhood of knowing they were not alone in their struggle to be therapeutic caring nurses. In sharing experiences through story and creative expression, Tori and her classmates vented; learned; gained hope; discussed problems; grew in confidence and perspective. Through what Banks-Wallace (1998) calls the 'emancipatory potential' of storytelling in a group, it was on the collective reflective level that a larger meaning of self and nursing was created.

According to Bohm (1985), dialoguing implicitly involves close listening and a tacit understanding of each other, despite unique experiences. He argued that dialogue is about finding meaning, not necessarily truth. In listening to the poetry and viewing the art, classmates urged further reflection by asking such questions as 'What does that mean?', 'What happened?', 'How did you feel?' These were not questions to prompt analysis, in the sense of tearing apart to see the details, but rather a linking of the different aspects into a whole. Prompted by the powerful images in the poems and drawings, reflective discussion provided opportunity for the emergence of a collective meaning of nurse-self, beyond what occurred through personal reflections. Isaacs (1994) calls this process 'creativity in the container'. Tori came to know herself better in context with other nurse-students.

Sharing at this level of openness and depth was emotional. Outward release of emotions through tears and laughter was testimony to the personal involvement the process encouraged, which has been strongly linked to increased learning (Brookfield, 1990). Within the level of collective reflection, it was the emotional bonds that made the process therapeutic. Mezirow (1991) argues that adults learn validity of their actions and ideas through others' confirmation. Such sharing engendered a pride in being a nurse and a hopeful feeling that there were other nurses who genuinely cared. Students inspired each other to look more critically at their caring, to be more aware of their patients, and to be better nurses.

Each level of reflection appeared to be necessary building blocks for the next level. Each level fostered what Johns (1998a) calls 'reflective cue' questions. The process prompted Tori to continuously shift her reflections from a narrow outward view to an inner perspective that was then brought to the surface again with a fuller understanding and wider perspective of self and practice. Although group reflective processing and support were the most vocalized need, it is important to note that Tori and fellow students would not have come to the circle so prepared to dialogue without having done personal reflecting before they arrived. Unexplored experiences do not provide insight. The reflective tools of story-writing (organizing the details) and poem and art-making revealed hidden details and feelings, which, in turn, increased personal insight and made the experience available for group processing.

Implications for nursing education

The understanding that is gained from this case study about personal knowing and use of therapeutic self has several implications for nursing educators. First, assignments that encourage reflection on caring-self and practice should be combined with the cognitive nursing process. Furthermore, opportunities for small group work that encourage sharing on the affective level needs to be valued in terms of time allotment and role modeling. If students practice reflective processing and learn to value its benefits, hopefully they will carry it into practice.

Another significant implication of this case study is that the use of creative expression stimulated reflection on practice on a deeper level than the descriptive story process. This addresses what educators expect of reflective tools (Brookfield, 1990). In this case study, if the nurse-student had stopped at the story-writing stage and had not translated the story into some art-form, she would have missed an important step in personal knowing about her relational self. Reflective journaling, a common assignment in nursing education, is often used as a descriptive accounting of the student's day, without addressing feelings and relationships. Student's use of poetry and art to examine experiences offers an additional alternative to increase awareness of caring-self in a transpersonal sense. The hesitancy that nursing educators and students might project in not being comfortable with creating art can be dispelled by putting emphasis on the process rather than the product. Valuing and sharing the crafting of poetry and art in an open trusting environment will honor the very mettle of the process. Reflective practice that increases the development of caring-self is an essential component in preparing competent caring nurses.

References

Allport, G.W. (1955) *Becoming: Basic considerations for a psychology of personality.* New Haven: Yale University Press.

Argyris, C. & Schön, D.A. (1974) *Theory in Practice: Increasing professional effectiveness.* San Francisco: Jossey-Bass.

Atkins, S. & Murphy, K. (1993) 'Reflection: A review of the literature'. *Journal of Advanced Nursing*, **18**: 6, 1188–92.

Baker, C.H. (1996) 'Reflective learning: A teaching strategy for critical thinking'. *Journal of Nursing Education*, **35** (1), 19–22.

Banks-Wallace, J. (1998) 'Emancipatory potential of storytelling in a group'. *Image: Journal of Nursing Scholarship*, **30** (1), 17–21.

Bartol, G.M. (1986) 'Using the humanities in nursing education'. *Nurse Educator*, **11** (1), 21–3.

Beckerman, A. (1994) 'A personal journal of caring through esthetic knowing'. *Advances in Nursing Science*, **17** (1), 71–9.

Belenky, M., Clinchy, B., Goldberger, N. & Tarule, J. (1986) *Womens' Ways of Knowing: the development of self, voice, and mind.* New York: Basic Books.

Benner, P. (1984) *From Novice to Expert.* Menlo Park, CA: Addison-Wesley.

Benner, P. & Wrubel, J. (1989) *The Primacy of Caring.* Menlo Park, CA: Addison-Wesley.

Bergman, S. & Krant, M. (1977) 'To know suffering and the teaching of empathy', *Social Science and Medicine*, **2**, 639–44.

Bertman, S. (1991) *Facing Death: Images, insights, and interventions.* Worcester, MA: Hemisphere Press.

Bevis, E.O. (1989) *Curriculum Building in Nursing.* 3rd edn. New York: National League for Nursing.

Bevis, E.O. & Watson, J. (1989) *Toward a Caring Curriculum: A new pedagogy for nursing.* New York: National League for Nursing.

Bishop, A.H. & Scudder, J.R. (1990) *The Practical, Moral, and Personal Sense of Nursing: A phenomenological philosophy of practice.* Albany: State University of New York Press.

Bohm, D. (1985) *Unfolding Meaning.* Loveland, CO: Foundation House.

Breunig, K. (1994) 'The art of painting meets the art of nursing' in Chinn, P.L. & Watson, J. (eds) *Art and Aesthetics in Nursing.* New York: National League for Nursing.

Brookfield, S.D. (1990) *The Skillful Teacher: On technique, trust, and responsiveness in the classroom.* San Francisco: Jossey-Bass.

Buber, M. (1953) 'I and thou' in Herberg, W. (ed.) *The Writings of Martin Buber.* New York: World. pp. 43–62.

Carper, B.A. (1978) 'Fundamental patterns of knowing in nursing'. *Advances in Nursing Science*, **1** (1), 13–23.

Cassidy, V.R. (1996) 'Literary works as case studies for teaching human experimentation ethics'. *Journal of Nursing Education*, **35** (3), 142–4.

Chinn, P.L. (1994) 'Developing a method for aesthetic knowing in nursing' in Chinn, P.L. & Watson, J. (eds) *Art & Aesthetics in Nursing.* NY: National League for Nursing. pp. 19–40.

Cumbie, S.A. & Rutherford, S.R. (1994) 'Weaving aesthetics into practice: The use of aesthetic techniques in group psychotherapy with clients remembering repressed traumatic memories' in Chinn, P.L. & Watson, J. (eds) *Art & Aesthetics in Nursing.* New York: National League for Nursing. pp. 233–45.

Darbyshire, P. (1994) 'Understanding caring through arts and humanities: A medical/nursing humanities approach to promoting alternative experiences of thinking and learning'. *Journal of Advanced Nursing*, **19** (5), 853–63.

Darbyshire, P. (1995) 'Lessons from literature: Caring, interpretation, and dialogue'. *Journal of Nursing Education*, **34** (5), 211–16.

Davis, C.B. (1989). 'The use of art therapy and group process with grieving children'. *Issues of Comprehensive Pediatric Nursing*, **12** (4), 269–80.

Dewey, J. (1933) *How We Think*. Boston: Heath Publishers.

Dewey, J. (1934) *Art as Experience*. New York: Perigee Books.

Dewey, J. (1938) *Experience and Education*. New York: Collier Books.

Diekelmann, N.L. (1993) 'Behavior pedagogy: A Heideggerian hermeneutical analysis of the lived experiences of students and teachers in baccalaureate nursing education'. *Journal of Nursing Education*, **32** (6), 245–54.

Dulles, A. (1985) *Models of Revelation*. New York: Doubleday.

Estep, M. (1995) 'To soothe oneself: Art therapy with a woman recovering from incest'. *American Journal of Art Therapy*, **34** (1), 9–18.

Feen-Calligan, H. (1995) 'The use of art therapy in treatment programs to promote spiritual recovery from addiction'. *Art Therapy: Journal of the American Art Therapy Association*, **12** (1), 46–50.

Fox, J. (1997) *Poetic Medicine: The healing art of poetry-making*. New York: Jeremy P. Tarcher/Putnam.

Freshwater, D. (1998a) 'From Acorn to Oak Tree: A neoplatonic perspective of reflection'. *Australian Journal of Holistic Nursing*, **5** (2), 14–19.

Freshwater, D. (1998b) 'Transformatory Learning in Nurse Education'. Unpublished PhD Thesis. University of Nottingham.

Freshwater, D. (1999) 'Communicating with self through caring: The student nurse's experience of reflective practice'. *International Journal of Human Caring*, **3** (3), 28–33.

Freshwater, D. (2001) 'The role of reflection in practice development' in Clark, A., Dooher, J. & Fowler, J. (eds) *Handbook of Practice Development*. London: Quay. Ch. 4.

Gaut, D. (1983) 'Development of theoretically adequate description of caring'. *Western Journal of Nursing Research*, **5** (4), 313–22.

Gibbs, G. (1988) *Learning by Doing: A guide to teaching and learning methods*. Further Education Unit, Oxford Polytechnic, Oxford.

Gilligan, C. (1982) *In a Different Voice: Psychological theory and women's development*. Cambridge, MA: Harvard University Press.

Goodman, J. (1984) 'Reflection and teacher education: A case study and theoretical analysis'. *Interchanges,* **15** (3), 2–26.

Green-Hernandez, C. (1991) 'Professional nurse caring: A conceptual model for nursing' in Neil, R.M. & Watts, R. (eds) *Caring and Nursing: Explorations in Feminist Perspectives*. New York: National League for Nursing. pp. 85–96.

Gunby, S.S. (1994) 'The lived experience of nursing students in caring for suffering individuals: A phenomenological analysis'. Doctoral dissertation, Georgia State University, 1993. Dissertation Abstracts International B, 54/08. 4078.

Habermas, J. (1977) *Knowledge and Human Interests*. Boston: Beacon Press.

Harr, B.D. & Thistlethwaite, J.E. (1990) 'Creative intervention strategies in the management of perinatal loss'. *Maternal and Child Nursing Journal*, **19** (2), 135–42.

Heidegger, M. (1962) *Being and Time*. New York: Harper & Row.

Heron, J. (1981a) 'Experiential research methodology' in Reason, P. & Rowan, J. (eds) *Human Inquiry: A sourcebook of new paradigm research*. New York: John Wiley. p. 153–65.

Heron, J. (1981b) *Philosophical Basis for a New Paradigm* in Reason, P. & Rowan, J. (eds) *Human Inquiry: A sourcebook of new paradigm research*. New York: John Wiley pp. 19–35.

Higgins, B. (1996) 'Caring as therapeutic in nursing education'. *Journal of Nursing Education*, **35** (3), 134–6.

Holden, R.J. (1996) 'Nursing knowledge: The problem of the criterion' in Kikuchi, J.F. Simmons, H. & Romyn, D. (eds) *Truth in Nursing Inquiry* Thousand Oaks, CA: Sage. pp. 19–35.

Isaacs, W. (1994) 'Dialogue' in Senge, P.M., Kleiner, A., Roberts, C., Ross, R.B. & Smith, B.J. *The Fifth Discipline Fieldbook.* New York: Currency Doubleday. pp. 357–64.

James, W. (1929) *The Varieties of Religious Experiences.* New York: Modern Library.

Johns, C. (1994a) 'Guided reflection' in Palmer, A., Burns, S. & Bulman (eds) *Reflective Practice in Nursing* Oxford, UK: Blackwell Scientific. pp. 110–30.

Johns, C. (1994b) 'Constructing the BNUD model' in Johns, C. (ed.) *The Burford NDU Model: Caring in practice.* Cambridge, MA: Blackwell Science. p. 20–58.

Johns, C. (1996) 'Visualizing and realizing caring in practice through guided reflection'. *Journal of Advanced Nursing,* **24**: 6, 1135–43.

Johns, C. (1998a) 'Caring through a reflective lens: Giving meaning to being a reflective practitioner'. *Nursing Inquiry,* **5**: 1, 18–24.

Johns, C. (1998b) 'Opening the doors of perception' in Johns, C. & Freshwater, D. (eds) *Transforming Nursing Through Reflective Practice.* Malden, MA: Blackwell Science. p. 1–20.

Jourard, S.M. (1964) *The Transparent Self.* Princeton, NJ: Van Nostrand.

Lane, M.T.R. (1994) 'The power of creativity in healing: A practice model demonstrating the links between the creative arts and the art of nursing' in Chinn, P. & Watson, J. (eds) *Art & Aesthetics in Nursing.* New York: National League for Nursing. pp. 203–222.

Lanzara, G.F. (1991) 'Shifting stories: Learning from a reflective experiment in a design process' in Schön, D.A. (ed.) *The Reflective Turn: Case studies in and on educational practice.* New York: Teachers College Press. pp. 285–320.

Leininger, M.M. (1981) *Caring: An essential human need.* Thorofare, NJ: Charles B. Slack.

Leininger, M.M. (1985) 'Transcultural care diversity and universality: A theory of nursing'. *Nursing and Health Care,* **6** (4), 209–212.

Leininger, M.M. (1988) 'History, issues, and trends in the discovery and uses of care in nursing' in Leininger, M.M. (ed.) *Care: Discovery and uses in clinical and community nursing.* Detroit: Wayne State University Press. pp. 11–28.

Leininger, M.M. (1991) *Culture Care Diversity and Universality: A theory of nursing.* New York: National League for Nursing.

Leininger, M.M. (1995) 'Assumptive premises of the theory' in McQuiston, C.M. & Webb, A.A. (eds) *Foundations of Nursing Theory.* Thousand Oaks, CA: Sage. pp. 387–402.

Lynn, D. (1995) 'The healing through art'. *Art Therapy: Journal of the American Art Therapy Association,* **12** (1), 70–71.

May, R. (1973) *Man's Search for Himself.* New York: Dell Publishing (Delta Book).

May, R. (1994) *The Discovery of Being.* New York: W.W. Norton.

Mayeroff, M. (1971) *On Caring.* New York: HarperCollins.

McNiff, S. (1992) *Art as Medicine.* Boston: Shambhala Publications.

Metcalfe, S. (1990) 'Knowing care in the clinical field context: An educator's point of view' in Leininger, M.M. & Watson, J. (eds) *The caring imperative in education.* New York: The National League for Nursing. pp. 145–54.

Mezirow, J. (1991) *Transformative Dimensions of Adult Learning.* San Francisco: Jossey-Bass.

Miles, M. (1985) *Image as Insight.* Boston: Beacon Press.

Morse, J.M., Solberg, S.M., Neander, W.L., Bottorff, J.L. & Johnson, J.L. (1990) 'Concepts of caring and caring as a concept'. *Advances in Nursing Science,* **13** (1), 1–14.

Moyers, B. (1995) *The Language of Life: A festival of the poets.* New York: Doubleday.

Nehls, N. (1995) 'Narrative pedagogy: Rethinking nursing education'. *Journal of Nursing Education,* **34** (5), 204–210.

Noddings, N. (1981) 'Caring'. *Journal of Curriculum Theorizing,* **3** (2), 139–48.

Noddings, N. (1984) 'Fidelity in teaching, teacher education and research for teaching'. *Harvard Educational Review*, **56** (4), 496–510.

Noddings, N. (1986) *Caring: A feminine approach to ethics and moral education.* Berkeley: University of California Press.

Noddings, N. (1992) *The Challenge to Care in Schools.* New York: Teachers College Press, Columbia University.

Parker, M.E. (1992) 'Exploring the aesthetic meaning of presence in nursing practice' in Gaut, D. (ed.) *The Presence of Caring in Nursing.* New York: National League for Nursing. pp. 25–37.

Parker, M.E. (1994) 'The healing art of clay: A workshop for remembering wholeness' in Gaut, D. & Boykin, A. (eds) *Caring as Healing: Renewal through hope.* New York: National League for Nursing Press. pp. 135–45.

Parker, R.S. (1990) 'Nurse's stories: The search for a relational ethic of care'. *Advances in Nursing Science*, **13** (1), 31–40.

Paterson, J.G. & Zderad, L.T. (1976) *Humanistic Nursing.* New York: John Wiley.

Powell, J.H. (1989) 'The reflective practitioner in nursing', *Journal of Advanced Nursing*, **14**, 824–32.

Predeger, E. (1996) 'Womanspirit: A journey into healing through art in breast cancer'. *Advances in Nursing Science*, **18** (3), 48–58.

Roach, Sr. M.S. (1991) 'A call to consciousness: Compassion in today's health world' in Gaut, D.A. & Leininger, M.M. (eds) *Caring: The compassionate healer.* New York: National League for Nursing. pp. 7–17.

Roach, Sr. M.S. (1992) *The Human Act of Caring.* Ottawa: Canadian Hospital Association Press.

Saewye, E.M. (2000) 'Nursing theories of caring'. *Journal of Holistic Nursing*, **18** (2), 114–29.

Samuels, M. (1995) 'Art as a healing force'. *Alternative Therapies in Health and Medicine*, **1** (4), 38–40.

Sandelowski, M.J. (1996) 'Truth/storytelling in nursing inquiry' in Kikuchi, J.E. Simmons, H. & Romyn, D. (eds) *Truth in Nursing Inquiry.* Thousand Oaks, CA: Sage. pp. 111–24.

Saylor, C.R. (1990) 'Reflection and professional education: Art, science, and competency'. *Nurse Educator*, **15** (2), 8–11.

Schön, D.A. (1983) *The Reflective Practitioner.* New York: Basic Books.

Schön, D.A. (1987) *Educating the Reflective Practitioner.* San Francisco: Jossey-Bass.

Sheppard, L.C. (1994) 'Art and beauty as healing modalities' in Gaut, D. & Boykin, A. (eds) *Caring as Healing: Renewal through hope.* New York: National League for Nursing Press. pp. 102–110.

Silva, M.C., Sorrell, J.M. & Sorrell, C.D. (1995) 'From Carper's patterns of knowing to ways of being: An ontological philosophical shift in nursing'. *Advances in Nursing Science*, **18** (1), 1–13.

Skillman-Hull, L.E. (1994) 'She walks in beauty: Nurse-artists' lived experience of the creative process and aesthetic human care'. Doctoral dissertation, University of Colorado Health and Science Center, 1994. Dissertation Abstracts International-B, 55/05, 1809.

Sterritt, F.P.F. & Pokorny, M.E. (1994) 'Art activities for patients with Alzheimer's and related disorders'. *Geriatric Nursing*, **15** (3), 155–9.

Tanner, C. (1988) 'Curriculum revolution: The practice mandate'. *Nursing & Health Care*, **9** (8), 427–30.

Vaught-Alexander, K. (1994) 'The personal journal for nurses: Writing for discovery and healing' in Gaut, D. & Boykin, A. (eds) *Caring as Healing: Renewal through hope.* New York: National League for Nursing. pp. 150–63.

Vezeau, T.M. (1993) 'Use of narrative in human caring inquiry' in Gaut, D. (ed.) *A Global Agenda for Caring.* New York: National League for Nursing. pp. 211–21.

Vezeau, T.M. (1994) 'Narrative inquiry in nursing' in Chinn, P.L. & Watson, J. (eds) *Art and Aesthetics in Nursing.* New York: National League for Nursing. pp. 41–66.

Wagner, A.L. (1995) 'Unleashing the giant: The politics of women's health' in Boykin, A. (ed.) *Power, Politics and Public Policy: A matter of Caring.* New York: National League for Nursing Press. pp. 63–81.

Wagner, A.L. (1998) 'A study of baccalaureate nursing students' reflection on their caring practice through creating and sharing story, poetry, and art'. Doctoral dissertation, University of Massachusetts Lowell, 1998. Dissertation Abstracts International, 99-(05), 334. (University Microfilms Inc. No. DAO 72699)

Wagner, A.L. (1999) 'Within the circle of death: Transpersonal poetic reflections on nurses' stories about the quality of the dying process'. *International Journal for Human Caring*, **3** (2), 21–30.

Wagner, A.L. (2000) 'Connecting to nurse-self through reflective poetic story'. *International Journal for Human Caring*, **4** (2), 7–12.

Watson, J. (1988a) 'Human caring as moral context for nursing education'. *Nursing & Health Care*, **9** (8), 423–5.

Watson, J. (1988b) *Nursing: Human science and human care: A theory of nursing.* New York: National League for Nursing.

Watson, J. (1994) 'Introduction' in Watson, J. (ed.) *Applying the Art and Science of Human Caring.* New York: National League for Nursing. pp. 1–10.

Watson, J. (1999) *Postmodern Nursing and Beyond.* New York: Churchill Livingstone.

Whyte, D. (1994) *The Heart Aroused: Poetry and the preservation of the soul of corporate America.* New York: Currency Doubleday.

Young-Mason, J. (1988) 'Literature as a mirror to compassion'. *Journal of Professional Nursing*, **4**: 4, 299–301.

Young-Mason, J. (1995) *States of Exile: Correspondence between art, literature, and nursing.* New York: National League for Nursing.

Zamierowski, M.J. & Gordon, A. (1995) 'The use of creative art forms to enhance counselling skills of hospice professionals in dealing with the bereaved'. *American Journal of Hospice and Palliative Care*, **12** (1), 5–8.

Ziesler, A.A. (1993) 'Art therapy: A meaningful part of cancer care'. *Journal of Cancer Care*, **2** (2), 107–111.

PART III

THE RESEARCHER'S PERSPECTIVE

Dawn Freshwater

It is generally recognised that there is an overlap between the skills of therapeutic nursing and the skills of researching nursing. Field and Fitzgerald capture this relationship succinctly, saying that 'In order to learn to nurse in a therapeutic manner the nursing student needs to be able to appreciate and evaluate nursing research and to be able to discriminate in the choice of evidence to guide practice' (1998: 100). The choice of research evidence used to underpin the practice of nursing and in particular therapeutic nursing is the issue under consideration in the final part of this book.

Research is always carried out by an individual 'with a life and a *lifeworld,* a personality, a social context, and various personal and practical challenges and conflicts, all of which affect the research, from the choice of a research question or topic, through the method used, to the reporting of the project's outcome' (Bentz & Shapiro, 1998: 4). Hence the motivation for the research and of the researcher is *vital* to the research process; here I use the term 'vital' to signify the organic nature of practitioner-based research. With the increasing institutionalisation and industrialisation of research, researchers may find themselves engaging in it as a technical process, rather than a vital process 'like a cog in the wheel of the modern industrial apparatus' (Bentz & Shapiro, 1998: 5) without reflecting on its meaning and purpose for the researchers' practice. (For an in depth review of the significance of the researchers' motivation in the research process, see Braud & Anderson, 1998). How does one ensure that the research process remains a vital one? What are the appropriate methods within which to understand the nature of therapeutic nursing? According to Field and Fitzgerald, 'Therapeutic nursing necessitates an eclectic approach to research generally insofar as nursing generates a range of questions that are most suitably answered through different research perspectives' (1998: 99).

The reformulation of subjectivity in research in the past decade has resulted in researchers presenting less sanitised versions of the research process. Okely (1992), a feminist anthropologist, contests that in relation to the research process, so much of the self is involved that it is impossible to reflect upon it by extracting the self. Moch underlines this in describing her experience of undertaking research with breast cancer patients; she reflects: 'At times I wondered if I was first as nurse and then a researcher or first as researcher and then a nurse. Sometime the difficulty arose because of my experience as a mother, wife, midlife woman, or professor. In other words the researcher experience and all the reflection and struggle happened, in part, because of who I am' (2000: 7).

When viewed in the context of research, reflection means 'thinking about the conditions for what one is doing, investigating the way in which the theoretical, cultural and political context of individual and intellectual involvement affects interaction with whatever is being researched, often in ways difficult to become conscious of' (Alvesson & Skoldberg, 2000: 245). In this sense, research becomes an expansion of consciousness and a process of construction, deconstruction and reconstruction through reflexivity, requiring a dialogic relationship of sorts.

Chapter 8, written by Carol Picard, links the notion of research as expanded consciousness with the concepts of reflection and praxis, in which practice, research and education are integrated. Carol's unique slant is her use of creative movement and narrative as modes of expressing the self. Describing the use of dance in the research experience, Carol develops this idea in relation to therapeutic nursing, arguing for an embodied response to the patient's needs. Carol's Chapter furthers the notion of transformatory research, demonstrating how the researcher can facilitate growth and development in the research participants. Thus she highlights how using the self as a therapeutic tool for research, allows for the possibility of the research to become a therapeutic endeavour for all concerned.

Researchers utilising single in-depth case studies or long-term analysis of organisational members as their method of data collection in research, often become at least partial participants in the research process and as such fall into the category of ethnographers. This is in contrast to the qualitative researchers who rely on interviews or non-participant observation techniques, who, as Elsbach (2000) points out, are less involved. In this sense it is likely that ethnographic researchers encounter research as an experience that is transformative, that is to say that the research 'profoundly affects their personal and professional identities' (Elsbach, 2000: 56). As in Chapter 2 in which Roderick McKenzie discussed his own process of transformation through the process of autoethnography, so Tessa Muncey in Chapter 9 outlines her own experience of using biographical ethnography to understand her own and her students' experiences.

Much has been written about the awareness of qualitative organisational researchers in the research experience (Boje, 2001; Van Maanen, 1988; Sutton & Schurman, 1985). However, this awareness has invariably focussed on the issue of how subjective interpretations and personal bias has affected the findings of the research, rather than how the research has affected the personhood of the researcher. Tessa clearly articulates the impact of researching the deviant case study on her own personhood, articulating the close relationship between herself and the participants, through artefacts, anecdote and biography. Sutton & Schurman (1985) discuss the close relationship that qualitative scholars have with their participants (which is not unlike the relationship that nurses have with their patients). This, they contend, may have a strong impact on their self-perceptions, indicating the potential for transformation that is held within the research encounter.

Where nursing fails, the trend has been invariably to find someone to blame, a scapegoat. As Wright notes, 'identifying and dismissing the "bad" nurses is seen as resolving the problem' (1998: 111). Clinical Governance (DoH, 1998), the drive to continually improve patient care, proposes an NHS culture within which openness, accountability and acknowledging our mistakes and learning from them can be fostered. However, this is easier said than done for as Wright comments, 'For nursing practice to become holistic, healing and humane, i.e. therapeutic, it requires a fertile ground in which to grow' (1998: 113). Tessa's reflection on the deviant case or the 'bad' nurse presents an interesting addition to the Clinical Governance debate, particularly in relation to the idea of scapegoating and the development of therapeutic practice within a culture that too easily leans towards blame.

The final contribution to this part and to the book is made by Gary Rolfe. Gary's chapter takes us back to the beginning, perhaps, as he says, closing the circle. But whilst we may be back at the beginning, we are not back where we started. Rather like the T.S. Eliot poem, we find that 'the end of all our exploring, will be to arrive where we started and know the place for the first time' (1935: 23).

Just as the client-centred roots of student-centred learning have been heavily criticised as over-emphasising personal meaning, understanding and personal power without addressing the broader organisational, cultural and societal context within which the individual finds themselves, so research, which uses the self as the main instrument of data collection, is also criticised by writers associated with the traditional positivist research paradigm. In deconstructing the dominant discourses in nursing research, Gary's chapter outlines a movement from suppression of self and objectivity in research to immersion of the self, where even subjectivity doesn't exist. Concerning himself with the repopulation of the research text, it appears that Gary challenges the reader to step out of the usual taken-for-granted cultural roles and values associated with research, and develop a resistance to enculturation (Maslow, 1987). Chapter 1 volunteered the postmodern sceptical position regarding the nature of the self, and in the final chapter Gary also provides a view from the edge. Commenting as he does on the clichéd and overused notion of using self as a research tool, forced me to revisit the term 'therapeutic use of self' and reflect further upon its meaning as the book comes to a close. I was left with the idea of integration, which Gary muses on, concluding that 'excluding the self from the research process, the roles of the researcher, practitioner and educationalist are kept irretrievably separate.' The aim of this book has been to illustrate the impossibility of such a separation for effective therapeutic nursing; but this is not just integral nursing, but nursing practised with integrity.

References

Alvesson, M. & Skoldberg, K. (2000) *Reflexive Methodology*. London: Sage.

Bentz, V.M. & Shapiro, J.J. (1998) *Mindful Inquiry in Social Research*. California: Sage.

Boje, D.M. (2001) *Narrative Methods for Organisational and Communication Research*. London: Sage.

Bradbury, H. (eds) *Handbook of Action Research*. London: Sage. Ch. 10.

Department of Health (1998) *Clinical Governance: Quality in the new NHS*. London: DoH.

Eliot, T.S. (1935) *Little Gidding. In Four Quartets*. London: Faber & Faber.

Elsbach, K.D. (2000) 'Six stories of researcher experience in organisational studies' in Moch, S.D. & Gates, M.F. *The Researcher Experience in Qualitative Research*. California: Sage.

Field, J. & Fitzgerald, M. (1998) 'Therapeutic nursing: emerging imperatives for nursing' in McMahon, R. & Pearson, A. (eds) *Nursing as Therapy*. Cheltenham: Stanley Thornes.

Maslow, A. (1987) *Motivation and Personality*. 3rd edn. New York: Harper and Row.

Moch, S.D. (2000) 'The researcher experience in healthcare research' in Moch, S.D. & Gates, M.F. (eds) *The Researcher Experience in Qualitative Research*. California: Sage. Ch. 2.

Okely, J. (1992) 'Anthropology and Autobiography: participatory experience and embodied knowledge' in Okely, J. & Callaway, H. (eds) *Anthropology and Autobiography*. London: Routledge. Ch. 1.

Sutton, R.I. & Schurman, S.J. (1985) 'On studying emotionally hot topics: Lessons from an investigation of organisation death' in Berg, D. & Smith, K. (eds) *Clinical Demands of Research Methods*. California: Sage. pp. 333–49.

Van Maanen, J. (1988) *Tales of the Field: On writing ethnography*. Chicago: Chicago University Press.

Wright, S. (1998) 'Facilitating therapeutic nursing and independent practice' in McMahon, R. & Pearson, A. (eds) *Nursing as Therapy*. Cheltenham: Stanley Thornes.

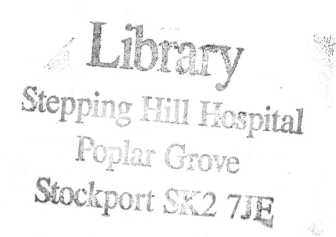

8 A Praxis Model of Research for Therapeutic Nursing

Carol Picard

A major contribution to nursing research from Margaret Newman (1999) is identifying praxis as the point where practice and research converge. Her theory of health as expanding consciousness and the nursing role of engaging in dialogue with persons to identify their patterns of relationships, is at the heart of a praxis approach to care. Newman (1994) described a reflective framework for praxis methodology, with two aims. The first is to support pattern recognition and the second is to advance the discipline by sharing findings with the larger nursing community. This chapter describes the use of Newman's praxis methodology, with the addition of creative movement as a source of expression of the person's story/pattern. This mode of expression holds potential to extend our theoretical understanding of health as expanding consciousness as people express meaning in an embodied form.

Health as expanding consciousness

According to Newman, health is expanding consciousness (1999). She defined consciousness as the capacity of the person to interact with all aspects of their environment, including other people. Each person has a unique pattern of engagement, which is expressed in what they identify as most meaningful. Pattern, according to Newman, is unique manifestation of the whole. Pattern is a qualitative dimension, different from quantity, and pattern recognition is an understanding of the shape that meaning takes over time. This pattern is what the physicist Bohm (1980) called the 'explicate order'. This order arises from an unseen, essential or implicate pattern of the whole of the person. As people recognize their pattern, they have an opportunity for growth through awareness. The capacity for self-reflection and self-understanding are aspects of expanding consciousness.

Using Young's theory of evolution of systems, Newman (1994) explicated stages of expanding consciousness from potential freedom to absolute freedom. At early stages, a person's consciousness is bound, as in young children. Most decisions are made for the child, until they begin to develop a sense of self. As a person self-identity develops, consciousness moves toward the centering stage. At this point rules are followed, but there is a focus on shifting away from the authority of others. As consciousness further develops, people come to what Newman calls a 'choice point', where old rules no longer apply and the need for

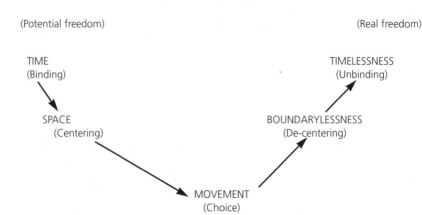

Figure 8.1   *Newman's basic concepts and Young's stages of evolution of
consciousness*
(*Note:* From *Developing Discipline: Selected
Works of Margaret Newman A* (p. 132) by Margaret A. Newman
(1995) New York: National League for Nursing. Copyright
1995 Margaret A. Newman. Reprinted with permission.)

self-awareness is heightened. This is the reflective turn in consciousness, and
making choices becomes more deliberate. The person can no longer rely primarily on rules or the experiences of others to guide them. Much like the hero's journey, the meaning and purpose of life becomes central and the person claims
authority for the choices they make (Frank, 1995). The stage of de-centering
involves continued movement towards growth and higher levels of freedom and
dedication to something beyond the self, often service to others. This again parallels the hero's journey of returning from a quest and sharing the wisdom of the
quest with others. The person has an awareness of their consciousness as extend-
ing beyond physical boundaries, conceptualized as transcendence. There is a
richer sense of connectedness with one's world and less of a need to control or follow prescribed rules. Transcendence is the experience of moving to a higher level
of consciousness, which is expressed in more meaningful relationships and greater
spiritual freedom (Newman, 1994). In the stage of unbinding, the sense of unity
with one's world is paramount and consciousness again broadens. Figure 8.1
depicts this evolutionary process as Newman has described it.

Health is a unitary transformative experience, which evolves in one direction
over time. In Newman's theory, health and illness are aspects of a unitary process
and not mutually exclusive. For example, a person may experience an illness,
such as cancer, while identifying meaning within the experience and be transformed in the process (Baron, 2000; Endo, 1996; Moch, 1990). According to
extant research in the experience of health within illness, it is often illness, loss
or the process of uncovering one's pattern which brings people to their choice

point and accelerates expanding consciousness. These life events are experienced as periods of disorganization, instability or uncertainty. Newman used the work of Prigogine and Stengers (1984) to illustrate how times of uncertainty and instability present opportunities for increasing complexity in self-organizing systems, described here as expanding consciousness. Reed (1991) has identified transcendence as an increasing sense of connection with one's self and one's world and a normative process in the oldest old. Her research also supports the Newman's belief that events that destabilize the person earlier in life might accelerate this process.

Nursing and expanding consciousness: the therapeutic use of self

Newman et al. (1991) identified the focus of the discipline of nursing as caring in the human health experience. Newman believed that caring is the moral imperative of nursing, requiring an opening of the heart to what she considers the highest form of knowing. She states: 'The health perspective demanded by caring is one of unconditional acceptance of the whole. The new rules call for unconditional love, which manifests itself in a sensitivity to self, attention to others and creativity' (Newman, 1994: 140). Newman also challenges the community of nurses to live caring both in practice and research. She did not make a distinction between the two activities, naming it praxis instead. The values of power and control are rejected, and she challenges nurses to practice within the unitary paradigm as a 'reflective, compassionate consciousness' (Newman, 1999: 37). It is in the nurse's capacity to be fully present to the patient that this compassion is expressed. Through dialogue and listening to a person's story of what is most meaningful, nurses can assist people to appreciate their pattern of connections in their world. For Newman, the development of insight into one's pattern supports expanding consciousness. People often seek nursing care when they are at a choice point in life.

Praxis is the therapeutic use of self, where the nurse lives the theory in practice. Praxis is the embodiment of the theory of health as expanding consciousness. The nurse appreciates the value of assisting the person to identify their pattern of connection to the world. The nurse also realizes that attending to her own consciousness allows him/her to create a healing environment for others. A praxis perspective means that theory is employed deliberatively and used in the service of transformation. The boundary between practice and research blurs. Practice as praxis is research in every clinical situation. At another level, the findings of this process can be structured and reported to the nursing community at large, through scholarly meetings and publications and have a greater impact on the discipline.

In preparation for nursing praxis, Newman suggests nurses attend to their own pattern of meaning, since appreciating one's own pattern and developing a reflective practice enhance the nurse's capacity to be fully present and notice the pattern of others. Like Watson (1999), she recommends a centering meditative practice to cultivate presence, first to self and then to others.

Movement and expanding consciousness

In the evolving nature of consciousness, movement is how a person experiences space and time. Movement is the fullest expression of consciousness and occurs in all orders of life organization, from the molecular to the universal (Zohar, 1990). The rhythm of movement promotes a sense of integration. Through movement, we come to know our world, others and ourselves.

Creative movement as artful knowing

Creative movement is an intentional artistic mode of expression of wholeness. Bauman (1999) invited nurses to examine art as a path of inquiry. Artistic expressions can cast light on to pattern, since art has the capacity to capture the essence of experience. When the essence of experience is illuminated, we are caught in an arresting awareness of the whole, of time and space and boundaries flowing together. Bohm (1998) referred to this as 'seeing deeply'. He believed that creating artistic expressions is the natural order. Dissanayke (1992) defines creativity as being open to this illumination of what was unable to be seen before. She believed art is a critical form of expressing meaning, of making the everyday special and of reinforcing shared significances between people. She demonstrated the universality of art-making as a mode of connectedness across cultures and believed that postmodern people are urgently in need of ways to communicate at this level with each other.

When people express themselves artistically through the senses, with deep meaning, it can expand consciousness. It is an opening of the heart, quite similar to Newman's definition of caring. Langer (1953) believed that art is crucial to the human evolution and a key way in which the expansion of consciousness occurs. Creative movement is a form of artful expression which I have incorporated into a caring praxis approach to understanding mid-life women. Gregory Bateson, a noted author on how persons come to know their world, suggested using different modes of expression to expand knowledge, stating 'Can I, for instance, change my understanding of something by dancing it?' (Bateson & Bateson, 1988: 195). Both creative movement and verbal expression contain roots of the implicate pattern. Since experience is an embodied process, exploring a bodily form of expression such as dance, can illuminate and uncover aspects of knowledge of the human experience (Halprin, 1995). Such embodied expressions are another mode of storytelling. My research examines creative movement as a way to express meaning. It is this intention to create meaning which differentiates this form of movement expression from other forms of movement such as yoga, where the person is instructed on prescriptive ways to move. Investigations into creative movement may provide a basis for further exploration of movement as a mode of health promotion and as a therapeutic modality. For example, movement may reveal pattern reflective of expanding consciousness, which verbally-impaired patients could use to communicate with others, or for nurses to understand better these patients. Also, since movement is the most complete expression of the whole, its integrative aspect may be experienced as healing.

Creative movement and nursing praxis

Studies grounded in Newman's theory using nursing praxis to explore health have used the narrative as a way to capture meaning and support pattern recognition (Baron, 2000; Endo, 1996; Endo et al., 2000; Jonsdottir, 1998; Lamendola & Newman, 1994; Litchfield, 1999). I have used the narrative and creative movement as modes of expression of the whole in three studies (Picard, 2000a; 2000b; 2000c). In most other studies where creative movement has been employed, it was used as an intervention, with the focus on measurement of selected aspects of psychological health such as anxiety and depression (Heber, 1993; Goldberg & Fitzpatrick, 1980). Nursing research using intentional creative movement has been limited and primarily quantitative. The subjects were identified by mental health problem, such as self-esteem, morale or depressed mood, which were measured as variables and treated with a movement intervention (Goldberg & Fitzpatrick, 1980; Harden, 1989; Heber, 1983; Stewart et al., 1994). Elsewhere, the dance movement therapy literature has generated rich discussion of the healing and health promoting effects of dance movement over the past 25 years. However, a survey of dance movement literature revealed that most published writings are presented in the form of clinical reports or case studies. A more systematic approach to investigating this mode of expression is limited. Published studies have examined persons with psychiatric illness or chronic conditions, with an emphasis that has been on symptom reduction rather than a focus on identifying pattern of the whole (Beaven & Tollinton, 1994; Berger & Berger, 1983; Bond, 1994; Dibbell-Hope, 1989; Lavender, 1992; Franks & Fraenkel, 1991; Milliken, 1990; Westbrook & McKibben, 1989).

Extending Newman's methodology with creative movement

This study is based on Newman's (1994) protocol for research on health as expanded consciousness and incorporates the addition of a creative movement expression. In this phenomenological approach, the researcher embodies the theory. This differs from a strict interpretive phenomenological approach, which Newman considers inadequate for research as praxis. Rather, the *a priori* theory and the pattern expressed by the participant together illuminate an understanding of expanding consciousness. The research process is one of engagement in which the consciousness of researcher and participant are shared. This Newman describes as a hermeneutic dialectic, which I envision as a dance. It is the weaving of an understanding of theory that the researcher brings to the inquiry, with the understanding of experience that the participant brings. The process that unfolds is a mutual one, with each person having an area of expertise: the nurse an understanding of pattern, and the person seeking care/participation bringing their life experience. Within the process there is the potential for enhanced awareness on the part of both parties. A recent publication by Moch and Gates (2000) examines in detail the experience of the nurse researcher in praxis.

Being fully present to participants is essential. Since it is important for the researcher to be aware of her own pattern prior to engaging with the participants, I kept a journal to reflect on my own pattern, and kept a daily meditation practice throughout the research process. Other praxis studies used transcribed dialogues as data. The following also includes data generated from an intentional creative movement experience.

Design of praxis project: patterns of mid-life women

Since no published studies using Newman's theory had examined a developmental age group, I decided to explore the consciousness of mid-life women. Two in-depth interviews were held with each of 17 women, ages 40–65. In addition, the women participated in one three and a half hour creative movement group experience. The sequence of data collection was as follows: first interview, the group experience and a second interview. All data collection took place within a five-week time period for each participant. In the first interview, the women were invited to share what was most meaningful in their lives. The length of the interview depended on the participant, ending when they felt they had shared what was important, to their satisfaction. Interviews lasted from 50 minutes to 2 hours, with an average of 75 minutes. All interviews were audiotaped and transcribed. In the creative movement group, participants were divided into two groups for the creative movement experience. The group assignment was based on the order of their response to the flyer to participate; the protocol included a trust exercise series, the activity of the creative movement expression, and a closure exercise (Boots & Hogan, 1981). The trust exercises were important to create a safe space in which to explore the creative movement expression. Trust exercises began with a handshaking introduction while walking around the room for each person to make contact with everyone. This was followed by an exercise called 'walking blind', where one person led a partner around the room while the person being led kept their eyes closed. They were invited to pay attention to how they sensed the room without seeing, suggesting a tuning in to bodily sensations. This also provided an opportunity for connection with other participants. The couples then changed roles, and then changed partners until everyone had made contact with everyone else. At each pause in the activity, participants were invited to comment on the process. The third exercise was a group trust building, where each person was invited to stand within the circle of participants and keeping their bodies rigid, give their weight to the group, known as a 'trust fall'. The group would work together to support the person's weight. The fourth and last trust exercise was to use a piece of large paper and pencil to draw one's lifeline. The women were then invited to walk the line, as if it were drawn on the studio floor. These activities took about half of the studio time. Finally, participants were invited to reflect on what was meaningful in their lives and to express it in movement. After working on this expression by themselves, they were invited to share the creative movement with the group and describe what it meant to them. I did the same. These creative movement expressions were videotaped. The closure phase involved inviting the participants to share how they experienced the group and their own expression. A brief meditative exercise focusing on the breath ended the group.

Data analysis was ongoing. After the interview and group experience, the transcripts were read while listening to the audiotapes, and then re-read carefully several times, with key words and phrases of meaning underlined. All underlined statements were then collated and examined for their place in the narrative or pattern. Videotapes of creative movements were examined for meaning and overall movement qualities. Verbal data from the videotapes were also transcribed. Following examination of all data sources, a construing diagram was generated using each woman's own words to describe meaning over time. Finally, I would create a piece of reflective art which captured in symbol how I understood their pattern.

Second interview

In the second interview, the researcher's construing diagram of pattern and reflective art was given to the participant for reflection and discussion. Each was invited to clarify or revise if something was missing or did not capture the essence of what was most meaningful. The researcher and participant also viewed the videotape of the creative movement. Participants were invited to reflect on the videotape, and the process as a whole.

Post-data collection analysis

Transcriptions of the second interview were then examined in the same manner as for interview one. Additions or corrections to construing diagram and/or artwork were completed. A narrative summary was generated to reflect understanding of pattern. Upon completion of data collection and examination of individual participants' patterns, the data were compared to one another for similarities and contrast. Data was then intensely examined in light of Newman's theory.

My understanding was expressed in construing diagrams, a pattern summary and a piece of reflective art shared with participants. Understanding was also reflected in the analysis of themes across participants and subsequent reflection on the theory of expanding consciousness.

Findings: meaning at mid-life

The women identified meaning in relationship as most important. Relationships included oneself, other people, a spiritual connection and nature. Each person identified challenges which were also catalysts for growth. These challenges were losses, illness and threats to relationships. Activities associated with the evolution of expanding consciousness beyond the choice point were choosing, balancing, accepting and letting go.

Relationships to self, other, spirit and nature

Relationship with oneself included taking time for self-care and reflection. Often this is had not been attended to earlier in life because of family obligations. Relationship to others involved a sense of being truly known to another as well as seeing others for their uniqueness. This connection was essential for wellbeing and expanding consciousness. Being known could occur at any time in life, but had particular significance for growth when present in childhood. For those who did not feel known, its absence made future relationships more challenging. The women recognized relationships as a mutual process of growth, often pointing to relationships with their children. A connection with the natural world was identified as restorative and a way to ground oneself in the world or universe. This was often also associated with a spiritual connection. The women often identified a deepening of their spirituality in which they incorporated religious traditions.

Loss, illness and threats to relationship: impetus for growth

These challenges were identified as choice points. Most participants had reached an important choice point by mid-life. These challenges were identified as valuable for growth and self-awareness. The value of suffering was expressed as 'no regrets' the source of learning about oneself, and acknowledging the good and the bad as making up the whole. Although each person's story and pattern was unique, the same elements were identified over their lives, but in differing time sequences. For example, one woman had experienced a choice point while caring for both of her chronically critically ill parents. She began to reflect on what held the most meaning for her, and had instituted better self-care and self discovery time instead of always being in service to others. Another person who did not feel truly known for her uniqueness as a child had such an experience in her thirties. What followed was a dramatic pattern shift in connection with other people as well. She shared that being known helped her to 'come out of the box I was in.'

Her creative movement was one of being huddled on the floor. She looked from left to right and in a gathering gesture, pulled first her right and then left hands towards her chest. Of this movement she said: 'This was, it was a softening of my heart. A letting-in of another person into my life to join me in celebrating being here.' Others who were late at coming to a choice point also experienced a rapid acceleration in connections once it had occurred.

Creative movement: opportunity for reflection and validation of pattern

The creative movement was experienced as integrative and holistic, and provided an opportunity for self-awareness and validated pattern. The experience was useful to some participants to draw on and continue to use even after the group was completed. Both the creative movement and the interview provided an opportunity for self-reflection. Many participants expressed valuing having enough time to tell their story and commented that although they found the process therapeutic, they appreciated the non-prescriptive approach to inviting reflection. In their words, it was not therapy but therapeutic. Participants, both in interviews and the group experience, valued being known and feeling accepted.

Exemplar: healing from abuse

Diane is a 42-year-old woman who grew up in an abusive household. Both her stepfather and her brothers were physically and sexually abusive to her, and she has had no contact with them since adulthood. No one in her family of origin honored who she was or connected with her at the level where she felt truly known. The message she received from her family was that she was not good enough. This pattern continued in her first marriage. Her husband constantly told her she was not good enough and exerted a great deal of control over her life and gave her no support. An example described by the participant as a lack of support was when she was recuperating from cancer surgery and receiving chemotherapy treatment. Her husband left her alone for 9½ months, taking their new baby and older child with him, to live with his mother.

In her mid-thirties, Diane began to have a sense of the possibility of making choices for herself. She took courses in emergency medical technician training. Despite her husband's attempts to undermine her goal, she did succeed in working part-time as an EMT for a while. As she began to exert her independence in small ways, her husband's controlling behavior became worse. When a friend with young children committed suicide, Diane thought she was seeing what might be her own path if she continued in her marital relationship. She developed cardiac symptoms and anxiety and was unable to function at work. Her physician referred her to a nurse practitioner/therapist. This was a person with whom she felt known, understood and supported. Her choice point was in leaving her husband and, temporarily, her two children. She was able to secure an apartment and begin her education to become a nurse. Key to this experience was having people who she says gave her a push or took a chance on her – people who could truly see her as a person. The support helped her to reflect and take action:

> I've learned that I really had a lot more in me, than I ever thought I did. It took me a long time to find my voice. So I got ways to express how I was feeling about things. The old cliché had been 'everybody else makes the decisions and you do what they say. It took a lot of soul searching. I don't feel like I have to get somebody's approval all the time. I was looking for my mother's approval – well, my ex-husband's – I knew I couldn't get, but I was always looking for approval someplace else instead of me. I finally found it.

She was able to mobilize resources, become connected to the community, took college courses, found ways to finance getting a degree in nursing, and created a new home for herself so her daughters could join her. She had developed close friends, something which was almost impossible when living with her ex-husband. Recently she re-married, to a person who is very supportive and caring. She now expresses herself in poetry: 'I don't really think there's much structure in them, but they're intended to bring out feelings and hurts.'

Most important in her life at that time were her profession, giving to others, her new marital relationship and having good friends. She also valued having comfort in her life and making good choices. Diane took her new learning to her patients. By being sensitive to the experience of others, she believed she was able to give comfort, that thing she so recently had experienced in her own life. She tried to meet life without expectations, to be open to experience as a way of stretching herself. She was also open to new connections with people. An illustration she shared was caring for an older woman in the Emergency Room, who was screaming and incoherent. No one had tried to figure out the cause of the woman's distress, attributing it to Alzheimer's disease. When Diane entered the woman's space, she immediately noticed the woman's eyes. 'She looked like she was out of control, and you know, she was just babbling about nothing.' Diana quietly engaged the woman first with eye contact and then speaking softly to her, making a connection. She was able to assess that the woman had probably had a stroke and was aphasic. Like Diane, she needed someone to notice her distress and reach out to form a connection.

Diane's creative movement reflected the central elements of meaning in her story. She walked quickly to the center of the floor and met the gaze of the other participants. She then sat cross-legged on the floor with her upper body curled over. She rose to a seated upright position, and reached out to the right in an arc, using her whole upper body in a gathering motion. She then repeated the gesture on her left. In both sweeping gestures her arms brushed along the floor, taking in the space from front to back. She used both arms together in a sweeping gesture forward, and folded her upper body into the lowered curled-in position with head down. Then she rose again to an upright seated position and extended her arms with palms up in a sweeping gesture outward. She made use of near and far reach space, while remaining seated on the floor. She did not use her lower body. She said to the group: 'This is about comfort. This is my comfort level. I pull in what I need and I give back part of me to the world.' When she watched the videotape of her movement and reflected on the day, she said:

When you try to put the – your emotions in a very condensed type of perspective, it really takes a lot of thinking and a lot of looking inside. Actually it made me think a lot afterwards. I saw parts of things I didn't really – I knew were there, but really didn't take thought in and – because right after I left my husband and kids I was – I had this push out, but it was kind of like – flying around and not trust the land you feel comfortable in. And I guess I have found a kind of comfort place now I can really feel safe in. I feel like I can still grow, but yet, I can always have a place to come back to that I know I'm grounded there. And that's a good groundedness, not one like a weight; it's more like a cloud to lie down on. I got a realization of feeling it, and not just knowing it. It sort of came within inside of me: 'Look, it's there!' [She re-experienced feelings she thought were gone and had a profound insight on this.] You have to find a place in yourself for it and then grow from it – that was one of the things I realized when I went through that – you can't leave it behind – it's part of your life. It's what makes you *you*. I can still have those feeling but I don't fall from them. I can grow without rushing into things. I can look ahead, then make good choices.

I created a piece of reflective art for Diane, a bird flying out from a cage toward a nest in a large green tree. Written on the bars of the cage were the words 'Do as I say' and 'Not good enough'. When I shared this work with her she laughed and said 'Actually, it's interesting because I have a poem I wrote that is with birds. It's about, um, being grounded and then – it's interesting! The picture is really so – it's so funny cause it just – I do – I write these poems and the main one is about a bird.'

In light of Newman's theory, Diane's early pattern was that of binding, where her needs were sacrificed for others in the family. She did not feel anyone knew who she was as a unique person. There were very few choices. This binding continued in her marriage to an abusive man. The shift in consciousness from binding to centering began following the birth of her children and she pursued training as an emergency medical technician. As her husband's abuse escalated, her pattern was one of disruption and turmoil. She was able to tolerate a high degree of turmoil for 12 years before her pattern shift. She was able to move beyond this pattern, spurred by the loss of a friend to suicide and the care and understanding of a nurse/therapist.

Her relationships with her world became much more varied and complex since her choice point. The shift in pattern to choosing also relates to self-discovery and self-care. She has many more close relationships and was able both to give and receive in a deeper way. Her creative movement was reflective of this shift in pattern in the theme of connection, comfort and choice. The use of movement provided her with an opportunity for self-awareness and understanding of the wholeness of her experiences in a way talking did not.

In response to the praxis process, Diane related that she had told her story before in other settings such as therapy, and that she could remain more detached from past experience in words than in the other mode of expression, movement. 'I thought the whole thing was very good. I got a lot out of this. It starts you thinking about things you just put off thinking about.' Like others, she was impressed with the focus being one of acceptance: 'It was focused in a non-judgmental way.' The group process was also important to her: 'Everybody was saying they all wanted to see each other again. It was kind of interesting. They were all so into this emotion and the feelings that were attached to it, that they were feeling it all themselves.' Diane has continued in a follow-up study, meeting annually to come together with the other women in the movement group to create an expressive movement and to meet with me to dialogue about meaning. Her story and movement continue to be focused on a balance between her own comfort and her care of others.

Conclusion

Nursing praxis is a way of creating a space for participants to co-create knowledge with the nurse. It is also a way to generate knowledge for the discipline. The therapeutic use of self through presence grounded in nursing theory engages people in dialogue about meaning to support insight into pattern. This can be enhanced by additional modes of expression such as creative movement. The experience of moving to what is meaningful provides another pathway to insight as illustrated by the exemplar presented. The therapeutic use of self creates a healing environment.

References

Baron, A. (2000) 'Life meanings and the experience of cancer'. Unpublished doctoral dissertation. Chestnut Hill: Boston College.

Bateson, G. & Bateson, M.C. (1988). *Angels Fear: Toward and epistemology of the sacred.* New York: Bantam.

Baumann, S. (1999) 'Art as a path of inquiry'. *Nursing Science Quarterly,* **12** (2), 111–17.

Beaven, D. & Tollinton, G. (1994) 'Healing the split: a psychophysical approach to working with sexually abused teenaged girls'. *Physiotherapy,* **80** (7), 439–42.

Berger, L.F. & Berger, M.M. (1983) 'A holistic group approach to psychogeriatric patients'. *International Journal of Group Psychotherapy,* **23**, 432–42.

Bohm, D. (1980) *Wholeness and the Implicate Order.* London: Ark.

Bohm, D. (1998) *On Creativity.* London: Routledge.

Bond, K. (1994) 'Personal style as a mediator of engagement in dance: watching terpsichore rise'. *Dance Research Journal,* **26** (1), 15–26.

Boots, S. & Hogan, C. (1981) 'Creative movement and health: expressive dance'. *Topics in Clinical Nursing,* **3**, 23–31.

Braud, W. & Anderson, R. (1998) *Transpersonal Research Methods for the Social Sciences.* Califorina: Sage.

Dibbell-Hope, S. (1989) 'Moving toward health: a study of the use of dance-movement therapy in psychological adaptation to breast cancer'. Unpublished PhD Thesis. California School of Professional Psychology: Berkeley/Alameda.

Dissanayke, E. (1992) *What is Art For?* Seattle: University of Washington Press.

Endo, E. (1996) 'Pattern recognition in Japanese women with ovarian cancer'. *ANS,* **20** (4), 49–61.

Endo, E., Nitta, N., Inayoshi, M., Saito, R., Takemura, K., Minegishi, H., Kubo, S. & Kondo, M. (2000) 'Pattern recognition as a caring partnership in families with cancer'. *Journal of Advanced Nursing,* **32** (3), 603–610.

Frank, A. (1995) *The Wounded Storyteller.* Chicago: University of Chicago Press.

Franks, B. & Fraenkel, D. (1991) 'Fairy tales and dance/movement therapy: catalysts for change in eating disordered individuals'. *Arts-in-Psychotherapy,* **18** (4), 311–19.

Goldberg, W.G. and Fitzpatrick, J.J. (1980) 'Movement therapy with the aged'. *Nursing Research,* **29** (6), 339–46.

Halprin, A. (1995) *'Moving Toward Life.* Hanover: Wesleyan University Press.

Harden, J. (1989) 'Effect of movement group therapy on depression, morale and self-esteem in aged women'. *Dissertation Abstracts International,* **51** (05), 2286B (University Microfilms No. AAG9016893).

Heber, L. (1993) 'Dance movement: A therapeutic program with psychiatric clients'. *Perspectives in Psychiatric Care,* **29** (2), 22–9.

Jonsdottir, H. (1998) 'Life patterns of people with chronic obstructive pulmonary disease: Isolation and being closed in'. *Nursing Science Quarterly,* **11** (4), 160–66.

Lamendola, F. & Newman, M. (1994) 'The paradox of HIV/AIDS as expanding consciousness'. *Advances in Nursing Science,* **16** (1), 13–21.

Langer, (1953) *Feeling and Form.* New York: Scribner's.

Lavender, J. (1992) 'Winnicott's mind psyche and its treatment'. *American Journal of Dance Therapy,* **14** (1), 31–9.

Litchfield, M. (1999) 'Practice wisdom'. *ANS,* **22** (2), 62–73.

Milliken, R. (1990) 'Dance/movement therapy with the substance abuser'. *Arts-in-Psychotherapy,* **17** (4), 309–317.

Moch, S. (1990) 'Health within the experience of breast cancer'. *Journal of Advanced Nursing,* **15** (12), 1426–35.

Moch, S. & Gates, M. (eds) (2000) *The Researcher Experience in Qualitative Research.* Thousand Oaks: Sage.

Newman, M. (1994) *Health as Expanding Consciousness.* Boston: Jones & Bartlett.

Newman, M. (1995) *A Developing Discipline.* New York: National League for Nursing.

Newman, M. (1999) 'The rhythm of relating in a paradigm of wholeness'. *Image,* **31** (3), 227–31.

Newman, M., Sime, A. & Corcoran-Perry, S. (1991) 'The focus of the discipline of nursing'. *ANS,* **14** (1), 1–14.

Picard, C. (2000a) 'Pattern of expanding consciousness in mid-life women: creative movement and the narrative as modes of expression'. *Nursing Science Quarterly,* **13** (2), 150–57.

Picard, C. (2000b) 'Family member's experience of patients with bi-polar disorder'. Unpublished raw data.

Picard, C. (2000c) 'Pattern as process: A follow-up study of mid-life women using creative movement and the narrative as modes of expression'. Unpublished raw data.

Prigogine, I. & Stengers, I. (1984) *Order Out of Chaos.* New York: Bantam.

Reed, P. (1991) 'Towards a nursing theory of self-transcendence: deductive reformulation using developmental theories'. *Advances in Nursing Science,* **13** (4), 64–77.

Stewart, N.J., McMullen, L.M. & Rubin, L.D. (1994) 'Movement therapy with depressed inpatients: a randomized multiple single case design'. *Archives of Psychiatric Nursing,* **8** (1), 22–9.

Watson, J. (1999) *Postmodern Nursing and Beyond.* London: Churchill Livingston.

Westbrook, B.K. & McKibben, H. (1989) 'Dance movement therapy with groups of outpatients with Parkinson's disease'. *American Journal of Dance Therapy,* **11** (1), 27–38.

Zohar, D. (1990) *The Quantum Self.* New York: William Morrow.

9 Individual Identity or Deviant Case?

Tessa Muncey

I have spent most of my life pursuing an elusive desire to fulfil the academic potential I exhibited as a child. My educational progress was interrupted by an event that was subsequently to become the object of my research interest rather than just an episode that enhanced my motivation to succeed academically despite the overwhelming weight of evidence that conspired against me.

Under the umbrella of a nursing qualification I achieved what I believed was success in academic terms. I was both a District Nurse and a Health Visitor before engaging in a first degree in Psychology. This degree enabled me to enter nurse education where I subsequently completed a Master's degree in Women's Studies that started my questioning of conventional approaches to what knowledge is. A knowledge system that appeared to exclude the meaning of the lived experience of many people whose stories lie outside the contrived world of empirical research.

A craving to be included in the academic community culminated in a doctoral study that paradoxically marks the end of my need to conform. All of my discomfort with received wisdom is finding solace in answers from outside mainstream evidence. The paradigm shift that I feel is occurring in the world is reflected in the shift in my own views to find solutions in a range of ideas outside mainstream evidence.

It would be untrue to suggest that the long haul up the academic ladder has been a waste of time because it allowed me to understand how knowledge is generated and the power structures that are in place to perpetuate certain claims. Expert knowledge is socially sanctioned in a way that common sense knowledge is usually not and in various practices is accorded higher or lower status dependent on how it has been produced and who is saying it. These practices have as their central theme the rules of science: that is the desire for objectivity and the defining challenges of reliability and validity. Within these tightly constrained parameters a special language defines and delimits what is included and excluded. The scientific community illustrates this in the condemnation of authors who use the first person pronoun when describing his or her place in the research. So at the same time as learning the rules of the research game my own story became entwined with what I was reading and hearing, and I started to notice that the expert voices were not telling my story.

At a recent conference one of the keynote speakers, Marilyn Parker (author of Chapter 6) likened the world of research to a super highway. As I reflect on my journey I note how apt this analogy is. Super highways are straight, dull to travel on; they have strict rules of behaviour and are devoid of those idiosyncrasies that make country roads interesting. Most importantly they stride across the country by passing the lived experience of all the small towns and villages that eventually become ghost-like and neglected by lack of interest. Mainstream research appears to me to be like this, tied up in rules and conventions that make the results appear dull and flat and completely ignore the idiosyncrasies of the lived experience of the communities that it bypasses, so that in time their stories become at best forgotten and at worst untold. This chapter will use my journey of enlightenment to illustrate how the seemingly deviant case can challenge the existing discourse and give a voice to the world of meaning that may have been unheard. Just as the various strands in our biorhythms weave and twist, rise and fall, the various channels of my world of meaning has gradually taken shape linking together seemingly disparate areas of my life. A pattern has developed over the last few years whereby I go to conferences to present a paper on some particular aspect of my current research and then I seek out all the papers at the conference that I can attend that satisfy my personal curiosity. My real interest is in the topic of teenage pregnancy. I listen to the many and varied explanations put forward to explain its cause, its side effects and its solutions and I'm disappointed. Sometimes I'll ask a question, sometimes I feel too despondent to bother. After all, the research sounds so authoritative, the explanations put forward sound plausible and if adults know it is not a desirable state of affairs then it seems reasonable to problematise it. If the young mothers do not accept the solutions put forward, then isn't this just another symptom of their immaturity? The reason I am so interested in the subject is because that event which changed the course of my life mentioned at the beginning was a teenage pregnancy. I am a teenage mother. Grey-haired now and chronologically older but forever labelled as a misfit.

As a researcher I am fascinated by the studies that attempt to explain the reasons for and lived experience of the pregnant adolescent. I listen to those that advocate earlier sex education versus those who would encourage wider distribution of contraception. However, as someone who herself became pregnant at 15, I feel uncomfortable with the official versions of that experience. I find a fissure growing between what I feel is trying to inform my experiences of being in a world as a particular subject and the theoretical formulations that claim to account for my experiences. This Chapter describes the process of using autobiography in a polemical way in order to refute some of the received ideas and to suggest that adolescent pregnancy should be placed where it belongs in the paradigm of abuse. At the point where I felt confident to publish my account in order to challenge the research community, I was faced with having to justify my interest in a single individual in my doctoral studies. The second part of the chapter adds support to the notion that an individual can also be a very effective technique for exploring in metaphors the paradox that is nursing in the twenty-first century.

Individual Identity

Jung (1958) stated that man's aim in life is the achievement of psychic harmony between cultivation of the self and devotion to the outer world; sadly his ideas have been neglected in pursuit of models of behaviour that neglect the spiritual. Mainstream psychology has given us 150 years of expert's advice about everything from child rearing to improving our memories. Our so-called common sense has been gradually infiltrated with the knowledge of the expert. However, the harmony between the outside world and myself felt fractured when examined against this so-called expertise. The psychosexual and the psychosocial vie with the behaviourist and various combinations of the contribution of nature and nurture have been the extent of the debate. But have we been too concerned with the present and the recent past? What about the psychosymbolic structures that have been the mainstay of the Shamanic journey? Shamanism is nearly as old as human consciousness itself, predating the earliest recorded civilisations by thousands of years. People can be brought into contact with their journey by taking them to sacred sites around the world. In these places it is possible to enter into a personal dreamscape, although this is also possible by other routes. The purpose of the quest is to resolve the past, empower you to receive insights into your purpose and your future and to experience ancestral, archetypal intelligence as a living force.

The journey consists of stages. In the beginning is birth and the separation of the spirit from the body, the separation from innocence. Born into a family chosen for the purpose of my journey. Wandering among the people of my journey, I was seeking a truth that looked and felt like me. In this early part of the journey is also a kind of death, a separation from innocence. This is the archetype of the orphan. As an orphan one 'wanders with intent' seeking the truth. At all stages of the journey there is archival material to illustrate the path. This transitional stage can be traced through my school reports. At 10 it was noted that I was 'alert and lively, working diligently, producing good work, showing real promise, with obvious enjoyment and very competent.'

By 15 I was 'not doing my best work, making little effort, lacking concentration, had a most unpleasant attitude and showing serious signs of inattention.' A very special person wrote in a letter to my parents at the time, 'I keep thinking of Tessa and how sort of semi-grown up and yet frightened she seemed at my last visit. Not frightened of any outside danger but rather aware of the changing feelings within her. Adolescence is, I suppose, the most terrible of our ages. Beyond it, safely or with scars, the adult tends to forget it, putting it out of mind the way nature has of burying the unpleasant.' During this time my innocence died and the scars were etched deep within. Like a black virus pervading my soul. Outwardly I struggled but my attention wandered with the effort and this is what the world saw and, I thought, judged me by.

This part of my journey was the longest, ending only with the realisation of what my truth was. Keeping secrets is one way of protecting the truth but it takes a great deal of energy. As I explored my self, I realised that the enemy was within me and instead of punishing myself for being different I could incorporate that difference into my psyche and heal myself. As I passed from warrior to healer, the important stage in respect of autobiography is the point of rebirth. At this point of rebirth I no longer worry about the future, I know what I am becoming and that is an ancestor. The archetype of the ancestor is resolved to history, resolved to herself and the realisation that life isn't real until it has been told like a story.

The starting point of rebirth in my journey was one of the most liberating educational experiences as I underwent a Master's Degree in Women's Studies. Liberating in that here was a course actively encouraging me to take a multi-perspective view about all issues. For the first time I found people allowing me to express a view without telling me I was wrong or misguided. It was not wrong to be passionately interested in something simply because I had personal experience of it. Perhaps the deepest resonance was with one of the first articles I read in preparation for my dissertation.

Nursing Histories: Reviving life in abandoned selves was a film made by Marian McMahon that brought together aspects of her self that contemporary social theory thought fit to exclude. She wrote 'In realising that the authority of the theory I was reading excluded me, I gradually came to realise that it couldn't heal what needed to be healed.' For the first time I realised that we don't just learn from formal historical events but from subjective feelings and thoughts with which we experience the events of our everyday lives, and so it was that I started to examine why I had never felt a 'proper' nurse.

Shortly after completing this exploration of the constructed reality of the nurse, I found myself in a novel situation. Away from home, in a foreign country, with only a friend and colleague for company, I found myself revealing parts of my life story that I had never told. Why was I still struggling, she asked when it appeared I didn't need to any more. It occurred to me that the social construction of mother was just as unreal to me as the artificial construction of the proper nurse. In my way I was struggling to understand the confusion I felt of living in a world as a particular subject and the theoretical formulations that claimed to account for my experiences just as McMahon had. The next stage seemed to be to examine this confusion. And so I took the opportunity to examine my life as a story. This opportunity came when a colleague was thinking of putting together a book on sexuality. I asked if I could contribute a chapter on teenage pregnancy, which was slightly different. It was a cathartic writing experience which was pivotal in changing my attitude to writing, culminating in a real interest in the stories of other individuals.

As the purpose of this chapter is to outline the process of using autobiography rather than the content so briefly, I took Graves' poem *Broken Images* to provide the theme for a consideration of the reasons for adolescent pregnancy, starting with my autobiographical account. The patriarchal child-rearing expert has portrayed an image of childhood that assumes relevance to everyone and provides a powerful catalogue of facts on which successful child-rearing should be based; mother-blaming being the ultimate sanction when things go wrong. As a feminist I mistrust the images and question the facts and their relevance given the hegemonic power they endorse.

I consider the argument that early unplanned pregnancy is not just a matter of failed contraception or lack of sex education advice but is part of the wider debate on childhood sexuality. I use my story to illustrate my discomfort at some of the well-documented explanations that are put forward to explain it. Briefly, this story consists of the events surrounding the birth of my son and in the publishing of the story I reduce it to a case study that briefly encapsulates the views of the key actors in the event.

Case study

On April 22nd a young woman was told that her pregnancy test was positive. She underwent a completely uneventful pregnancy, which culminated in the birth of a very healthy baby boy on December 14th.

The girl was 15 years old. The midwife condemned her as a 'promiscuous young woman who failed to use contraceptives'. The social worker appointed to advise her said 'just give him up for adoption and get on with your life'.

The father of the child was arrested but not charged with unlawful sexual intercourse.In an informal autobiography 23 years after this event, the girl's mother presented her with 'The Grandmother's Tale'. In it she had used her many talents to pass on fragments of her life. Photography, pressed flowers and calligraphy adorned a text that conjured up happy days amidst the pleasures of the countryside. Wild flowers, walks, cycling all unfolding with a rosy glow of retrospection. Even the war set against the backdrop of the delights of new countryside when evacuated to a first teaching post in Worcestershire. However, she reports that:

> The 12 years of country plenty were followed by 10 leaner one's back in town – out of our natural element perhaps, so many things seemed to go wrong. But it was not to be forever; we decided to move and looked around for a new country cottage.

In those 10 lean years the girl was subjected to repeated incestuous sexual abuse. Her confusion increased, her self-esteem plummeted, she felt unable to tell anybody. Nobody seemed surprised when after a very successful junior school education she started to fail at school. Sex became the currency of affection and nurturing; she glided effortlessly from sex at home to sex with others. Nobody asked the right questions that might have elicited the real problems. School blamed her for failing there. Family were content to let the early pregnancy be blamed as adolescent ignorance. What none of them saw was the bleak and twisted world of a girl whose self-esteem was so blighted by her experiences that the idea of a baby to care for was, in a naive way, a treat to look forward to. A girl for whom sexual practice had been a reality for years. The unspeakable kind of incestuous relationship about which there is no one to confide in (Muncey, 1998).

It is perhaps interesting to note that this case study was anonymised at the suggestion of the book's editor, who perhaps rightly or wrongly decided that the story was best concealed in this way. To protect who, is not quite clear but other reactions to telling the story suggest that the victim or survivor's stories are often hidden this way in the media as well as the literature. This could have the effect of sanitising the work and almost certainly loses the powerful impact that anonymity conceals. In a critique of the literature by a health professional, the main features of the views about teenage pregnancy are deemed to be:

1 The young pregnant adolescent is not only held responsible for the moral decline in society, particularly the threat to the nuclear family, but deliberately acts to obtain welfare benefits by deception.
2 Sex education paradoxically encourages sexuality in the innocent, happy child and yet lack of it increases the likelihood of pregnancy.
3 Adolescent pregnancy carries considerable health risks and causes educational failure and poverty.

This chapter is not about this critique but the process of publicising an account that contradicts or adds another dimension to the story of teenage pregnancy. An account that suggests that the myth of childhood happiness/innocence and early forced sexual intercourse be explored in the discourse about early pregnancy. The obvious question to me is not why do young girls get pregnant, but why do they engage in sexual behaviour? So leaving aside the considerable gaps and anomalies in the literature, I will move on to the reaction to this published account.

After the story

If my story has anything to add to the debate about teenage pregnancy, to enable my colleagues and other interested parties to negotiate care with these young women successfully, then the reaction of these people would be vital to the process. If my voice was to take its place in this particular world of meaning, then it would have to be received and valued for it's contribution. Following the publicising of my story I have continued to attend conferences and engage in debate. The results suggest that my story does not fit neatly with the received view of the professionals and researchers. At conferences I continue to hear these voices. One such study in the Tyne Tees area of England was setting out to consider why the rate of teenage pregnancy in that area is the highest in the country. The research team planned to go out amongst the young women and ask them. Isn't it interesting, I pointed out, that several years ago a certain Dr Marietta Higgs was castigated for suggesting that in this same region child abuse was rife? Did they think the two could be connected? They hadn't, but concluded that it was a very interesting point. However, it might be too difficult to investigate! Pregnancy can't be kept a secret but incest can.

The other intriguing result of using autobiography is that some people will still refuse to believe it. One of my students chose the topic of teenage pregnancy on which to perform a critique of research literature. I suggested she might be interested in reading the chapter I had written. It was duly read and returned to me with a cursory note suggesting that however interesting my view I hadn't, in fact, put forward an explanation about teenage pregnancy, I was discussing sexuality which was quite different. This healthcare professional was not alone in this viewpoint. When discussing the topic for a conference paper on an autobiographical approach to teenage pregnancy to a group of research students, I outlined the gist of my argument based on my personal experience, namely that teenage pregnancy should be placed in the paradigm of abuse. One group member was adamant that I was wrong. She knew that the two were unconnected, in effect suggesting that I was either a liar or that my own story was so far removed from the 'truth' as to be worthless.

It therefore shouldn't be a surprise that the idea doesn't have many supporters if a real account is met with disbelief. Last year I read a letter in a national newspaper suggesting that girls left school with babies instead of GCSEs because their mothers colluded with them to produce a child to fill the gap of the empty nest; the name of the author was clearly stated. My reply outlining the sentiments of my view was anonymised despite not having asked it to be. This raises questions about the use of sensitive stories in research, but rather than hiding them, raises challenges about how to respond to them sensitively. In the light of these reactions I would emphasise the need for personal safety in the journey. As previously stated, anonymising the story is one way, but strengthening one's resources with both professional help and carefully selected individuals whom one can trust, is vital.

Analysis, at its best, begins every session with three convictions: each person has a story, their story makes sense, and the story is worth listening to. I know there are many valuable stories to be told. I believe that autobiography is a way of entering the personal dreamscape. I was a long time finding a writing style that was comfortable. After the children left home I started creative writing classes. Sally Cline* told us that 'writers are people who write', not specially assigned individuals but people like us, if we wanted to. In a short space of time I found my own style combining the personal and the public, the anecdotal with the theoretical.

'Polemic' means controversy, discussion. Its etymology is from the Greek, *polemos* meaning war, disputatious, argumentative, fond of debate, contentious. Autobiography is in Jungian terms the balancing of the four psychic functions. The bringing together of feeling, intuition, sensation and thinking into a quadrated world, a fourfold structure of equilibrium and depth. If an autobiography is to be truly polemical, I believe these four functions need to be brought together in order to continue the debate.

To add strength to the debate I continue to seek others who are telling a similar story. It would appear that unless you have a very particular type of trusting relationship with the young people themselves, asking them about their lives at the time the pregnancy occurs will not necessarily elicit the whole story. For reasons to do with power and fear and lack of support, most young people will tell the story that best fits the received view. It is not until they reach a stage in their lives when they feel safe or work with someone whom they can trust implicitly can the story be safely told. One of the key features of self-reflection is the need to have the freedom to make a genuine choice. If a difficult part of the journey is to be described without fear it is likely to be at the point of rebirth. It is not possible to ask young girls to reflect on the experience they are currently engaged in.

In a society that puts teenage pregnancy in the same discourse as problem, there is no room to discuss the benefits of such an experience. There is also no room to consider what else the discourse of teenage pregnancy could contain. In denying my story from the evidence-based world of healthcare I realise that the rest of the story is also missing. If asked for a title for my autobiography I would probably say 'A single mother who happens to be married' because for me the well-documented problems of the young mother were not mine. I did not get pregnant to gain welfare benefits by deception, I have not been an economic drain on society and I have not remained uneducated. What has been a problem, though, as I'm sure it is for many girls who get pregnant at an early age, is that I did not stay in the relationship with the child's father. This has meant that in order to maintain a further relationship I have entered the world of reconstituted family life. If a researcher were to ask me what the problems of being a teenage mother were, my answer would be quite simply step-parenting. Trying to balance the needs of someone else's child within a relationship is extremely difficult. There is an abundance of evidence that points to this being a problem where second and subsequent relationships break down, where children are abused by step-parents. This is a story that isn't told in the same discourse as teenage pregnancy and requires a different research stance. The story needs to be told at a different time and in response to different questions, and most importantly the teller needs to be the mother herself at whatever stage on the journey it is safe to disclose.

Deviant case

At this point in my story I was grappling with the academic world's perception of proper research. I could already see that there were parallels between case study research I was attempting to do and contemporary ethnography wherein autobiography as a technique fits in. They can both draw on multiple methods in an attempt to understand the meaning behind the actions and beliefs of those they study. Both stances raise serious questions about the effect of the researcher on the outcomes. On the one hand, the researcher may use reflexivity with regard to their participants using self-awareness to enable them to be conscious of the likely effects that they may have on the results. Alternatively, if the researcher acknowledges that she is an integral instrument within the study, this inside knowledge could be used to strengthen the interpretations.

This second half of this chapter juxtaposes my own journey of self-discovery with one voice from a doctoral study attempting to consider the notion of the good nurse and the implications of this for selection and retention of nurses (Muncey, 2000). I will argue that if researcher and participant are in the same universe of discourse, deeper understanding of nursing metaphors will be demonstrated. Metaphors are one way in which ideological ideas are found in language. Using one interview with a student nurse, two metaphors were elicited: 'nurse as rescuer' and 'nursing as reparation for disease'. It will be argued that these metaphors are not congruent with current healthcare policy which seeks to promote health and encourage independence rather than to act as handmaidens to curers of the sick.

When I started my doctoral studies, I set out to do what many researchers do and that is to discover answers to large questions using a variety of methods to satisfy the PhD examiners. Along the way, my feelings about research changed. As already stated, I saw a pattern emerging whereby I would go to conferences to present a paper on some particular aspect of my current research and then seek out all the papers at the conference that satisfied my personal curiosity, namely teenage pregnancy. This started my interest into personal meanings of events and behaviours that are not generated by mainstream research and led me into the world of autoethnography and the idea of the deviant case.

At the beginning of my research I set out to investigate various images of the 'good' nurse, identify core common characteristics associated with a good nurse, and determine areas of appropriate personal development and support that could be incorporated into the general training of nurses for the twenty-first century. The Clothier Report (1994) into the Allitt affair prompted this research and my interest in the subject reflected my academic interest in psychology and my professional interest as a nurse teacher.

The experience of being a personal tutor responsible for supporting student nurses for 13 years had highlighted that many of them endure emotional disorders during their training such as anxiety attacks, eating disorders and depression. These disorders are associated with low self-esteem and are usually associated with dysfunctional family backgrounds (Yates & McDaniel, 1994). Rew (1989) suggests that nurses may comprise a subset of young adults who have histories of childhood sexual exploitation and who exhibit symptoms of low self-esteem and depression. Nurses who overcome their problems and develop self-awareness can contribute to patient care with increased empathy (Kenny, 1994). People with low self-esteem seem to be attracted to nursing because of the gain in personal reward that results from caring. (Barker et al., 1996; Yates & McDaniel, 1994) The nurse–patient relationship has a power balance that enables the nurse to maintain personal control at work that she may not have in her personal life.

However, towards the end of the study I found myself narrowing down the focus of my interest. I went from nurses in general to one cohort in particular and then selected 12 students for in-depth interviews. It was while focussing on the analysis of these interviews that one student was drawn to my attention for particular scrutiny. It was not an example of a good nurse who seemed obvious to spot as someone with high self-esteem, good assertiveness skills and an internal locus of control, but the behaviour of one student who just did not seem to fit. I started to think about my experience of meanings in nursing practice. I remembered that early in my district-nursing career I had a salutary lesson in the meaning of disease to a patient that was at odds with the medical model employed by the health service. A lady in her eighties with chronic venous ulceration to her legs underwent a radical programme of management of her leg ulcer that resulted for the first time in many years in the ulcerated areas becoming healed.

As a new and keen district nurse I was very pleased with the progress and was puzzled by the patient's increasing anxiety as the ulcer healed. Anticipating that her anxiety was related to the proposed end of the nurse's visit, I reassured her that occasional visits would be necessary to reassess the condition of her legs following recovery. Also that she could be put forward as someone who may benefit from a regular visit from a local sixth-former. Nothing would placate her and in exasperation one day I asked her what was worrying her so much. She very sadly told me that for years she had seen a regular discharge from her leg which she had decided was her body's way of rejecting 'the bad' from her body. If it was now healed, she was very concerned that this same 'badness' would continue to circulate around her body. In assuming that we shared a common view of the physiology of the body, albeit fairly limited on her side, I had failed to ask the relevant questions that got to the heart of the problem.

Deviant case analysis

It occurred to me that the meaning of being a good nurse was quite different to different nurses. On the one hand, there were those who wanted to be involved in curing the sick, who were fascinated by the medical model, and then there were those who wanted to promote individuality and tolerate difference and negotiate care with patients. Given the trends within healthcare, the latter is now the desired outcome and therefore needs to be encouraged. Whilst the primary aim of my research remained to identify characteristics associated with a good nurse, towards the end of the study it appeared that the negative characteristics could not be ignored if strategies for effective training were to evolve from the analysis. This may be particularly so as the inherent characteristics that students bring to the course play a key role in their development as nurses. Across-method triangulation has been used to establish the credibility of the case study, using qualitative methods to support the quantitative data (Begley, 1996). This is deemed to help with the completeness of the research findings and establish the credibility of particularly the qualitative data (Redfern & Norman, 1994; Nolan & Behi, 1995).

As a result of the huge amount of data generated by the interviews any analysis, even using the participants' own words, remains a small representation of the group's experience. As McCaugherty points out, 'rather like the average British family, who have 2.2 children and live in the middle of the Bristol Channel, the average patient is not often met' (1991: 1057). Just as there is not an average patient, it could be argued there is not an average nursing student. In selecting one student for detailed study, the purpose is to bring together the personal, scientific and experiential knowledge, the synthesis of which is referred to as professional judgement (Clarke et al., 1996) or expertise (Benner, 1984). In understanding the experience of one student, interventions that are more specific may result.

This left the decision as to which one case should be selected. Efforts had been made to leave an audit trail (Guba & Lincoln, 1981) throughout the study, but at this stage I followed a hunch that the deviant case would be worthy of detailed reading. Meleis (1991) maintains that theories evolve from ideas, which in turn are a product of, amongst others, hunches, intuitions and inspirations. This links in nursing to the idea of expert practitioners basing their judgements on intuitive knowing (Benner, and Tanner 1987).

Some of the most useful analytical phenomena are cases that seem to go against the pattern or are deviant in some way. In this type of work, deviant cases are not necessarily disconfirmations of the pattern (Potter, 1996). The deviant case can highlight exactly the kind of problem that shows why the standard pattern should take the form that it does. Three interviewees presented themselves as interesting possibilities. M was a particularly good example of positive nurse characteristics with high self-esteem, assertive behaviour and internal locus of control. She achieved the highest marks in the theoretical component of the course and whilst she was a challenge to teach there is no doubt that her success on the course had little to do with needing support from the facilitators. P struggled through the course and appeared to exhibit negative characteristics of external control and lack of assertiveness. However, his high self-esteem made him a popular student and his intrinsic motivation to succeed, like M, suggested that very little was required in the way of support apart from the provision of a range of resources. Ha, on the other hand, exhibited the whole range of negative characteristics, low self-esteem, lacking assertion and external control and was generally considered by students, lecturers and clinicians to be an outsider who appeared unaware of inappropriate behaviour. Ha, then, was a student for whom supportive interventions would appear crucial to successful development of positive nurse characteristics and was selected for further detailed analysis.

Nurse as rescuer of the sick

Throughout the study, Ha has consistently presented herself as a very troubled young lady with low self-esteem, poor assertion skills and a fixed view of nursing as an adjunct to medicine. She sees herself as a rescuer of patients and views the world of nursing as a myriad of technical skills and responses to diseased bodies. She completed the course, passed her theoretical and practical assessments, but remained quite aloof from the group. In selecting her interview for further scrutiny it can be demonstrated how deeply-seated her views were and just what might be needed to enable this person take on the attitudes and beliefs required to enable her to nurse into the twenty-first century in line with current nursing initiatives.

Kelly's (1980) principle of reflexivity puts researcher and researched in the same universe of discourse. His sociality corollary allows the researcher and the researched in this context to allow the construction processes of one person to play a role in the socialising process of another. This form of role taking is close to the concept of role taking originated by Mead (1934), which is the process by which an individual is able to imaginatively cast him or herself in the role of others and thereby anticipate their actions. In this understanding should come a clearer view of how this person could be helped to make the transition to a different view of nursing. Wetherell argues that in order to understand the 'relatively autonomous ideological practices of a culture' (1989: 89) it is important to

Table 9.1   *Nurse constructs from study one*

Reflective judgement	Rescuer
Facilitating, objective, rational, proactive, selects knowledge, creative problem solver, clear thinking, effective decision maker, thoughtful, questioning.	Imposes care, rescues patients, take over, automatic response, create problems, controlling, unquestioning, indecisive, not selective, equivocate, automated, clouded judgement.
Disengages from personal feelings	**Strong personal need**
Respects patients values, aware of strengths and weaknesses, advocate, consistent, caring for people, integrity, creates choice, accept secret world of patients, identify patients needs.	Selfish, unresolved life experiences, manipulable, overstep boundaries, detached, personal involvement, expose vulnerability, lacks integrity, restricts care.

consider what is thought of as common sense to the people within it. Interestingly, ideology which generally represents any system of ideas and norms directing political and social action is usually only used to refer to other's ideas which are perceived to contain falsehoods and distortions (Flew, 1989). So perhaps nurses refer to the ideology of medicine, which distorts the view of nursing, but not to 'new nursing' as an ideology. Evidence of ideological ideas can be found in language and 'linguistic repertoires are the substance which constitute these broad meta themes' (Wetherell, 1989: 90). They often present as metaphors such as in healthcare where, for example, doctor is usually viewed as father and nurse as mother.

There are two metaphors that recur throughout the interview:

- nurse as rescuer; and
- nursing as reparation for disease.

One response, which perhaps summarises Ha's two metaphors, is her response to what she feels proper nurses do:

> A proper nurse is someone who works in a hospital ... and cares for people ... ill people and I think I have got quite an empathy for ill people and perhaps there is a little bit about the power issue there, you know and they need me to help them get better.

Nurse as rescuer

In the bi-polar constructs of the good nurse in study one, two aspects are relevant to Ha's views (see Table 9.1). The rescuer with strong personal need is someone who will impose care and have a problem with boundaries.

In the interview, there are many examples that suggest that Ha has a problem with boundaries. She talks about personal and professional boundaries, boundaries between college and hospital and the need for clear boundaries in knowledge so that she can learn by rote. Throughout the interview she refers to herself as 'I' when she is referring to things she likes or wants or about relationships in particular, and 'we' whenever she refers to anything to do with students, practical things, changes, need to learn. This implies she has a clear view of herself as a person with needs and wants in terms of relationships but wishes to identify with the student body when considering her needs as a student nurse.

Personal and professional boundaries

Within her problems of defining personal and professional boundaries, she refers to her need for clear edges to be shown and the need for respect and trust.

> I think at first as a student you want to please everyone, your CPS, the staff on the ward and your patients but I do realise in life you are not going to please everyone and that should you know, you should accept with some people there's just going to be an individual difference between you and them and you should agree on keeping away from each other. ... I feel disappointed that I haven't pleased them and I feel that it is my fault why there is a problem in the relationship but I also believe if you're not going to get on then its best to leave it because you can make it worse by trying to, trying to be friends.

Whereas she defines a professional relationship as:

> ... one where you can agree to work with each other and do your job and do your best for the patient, fit in with the team, but then like if you have social events on the ward and like going out to the pub one night perhaps you won't decide to go.

Disclosure is another ingredient of boundaries that Ha is unsure about:

> ... knowing how much of yourself to disclose, I think that takes time and it is quite skilled ...

She then describes in detail a situation where she oversteps the boundaries and regrets it. She reveals something to a CPS, in a particular placement when she is upset, believing it to be confidential only later to find that it has been written in her assessment document. On being given the opportunity to remove the report, she chooses not to. Immediately following this revelation, she then describes an incident whereby she betrays the confidentiality of a young man, believing it to be best for him.

> I felt I did the right thing and I think deep down he knew I was going to go and tell someone and I think he told me because he wanted other people to know.

In revealing that she believes the patient confided in her so that she would report the matter, suggests she also thought revealing her feelings to the CPS may have brought to light an issue she was finding difficult and wanted it to come to the attention of her tutor. This may also explain why later in the interview she is disappointed that her relationship with her tutor is poor.

Ha mentions touch on three occasions, believing touch to be an essential ingredient of her relationship with patients, but this tends to contradict her boundary between personal and professional as she implies that touch is something that strengthens friendship with patients.

I like the touching but then that's my sort of personality … I believe that just touching someone and holding their hand reassures them as much as a long conversation.

… it is just a power thing, they're laying in bed and you're standing there 'I'm the nurse, I want you to do this' whereas if you get down to their level and touch them, its saying, you know, I want to touch you, I want to be friends.

Other boundaries that Ha mentions as problematic are the ones between college and hospital and the parameters of the knowledge she needs to acquire.

… at the moment it seems like it's the college and the hospital – there's a need to link the two.

She does not see herself as being able to initiate any of the relationships that she wants to have with either her link teacher or her personal teacher, believing that they have a responsibility to come to her and expressing a need to be pampered and a need to try and please everybody.

There is a definite sense of equating the student experience with that of a child who needs looking after and the day of qualification being the entry to the adult world, where suddenly she will assume responsibility for herself. She confesses she has difficulty communicating with children or anybody who makes her feel out of control, and cites an example of not being able to understand why people get drunk because of the lack of control it induces. She blames her own sociali-sation for these feelings. However, she hopes these will disappear with time.

Boundaries in learning

In expressing a desire to learn everything by rote, Ha wants clear boundaries to the levels of learning that she is required to undertake. Given her vision of nursing as a job to care for the sick, it is not surprising that she feels biology is helpful in enabling her to understand conditions and medication but wants to know exactly what to learn. She sees no relevance in social policy or the social sciences:

I like learning about conditions and taking the blood pressure because that is what I see a nurse as doing whereas lectures on social policy and some sociology lectures I can't quite see the direct relevance to nursing whereas when you have a lecture on taking someone's blood glucose I can see the importance of needing to do that in a clinical area.

This irrelevance is also related to the way in which Ha wants to learn by rote:

… if you gave me an exam on something like social policy I probably wouldn't do very well because I am not interested in it, I can't see the relevance so I wouldn't learn.

You can't learn psychology and sociology quite so easily but biology you can learn by rote and just spiel it back.

Nurse as reparation for disease

The second metaphor that is present in Ha's words is the linking of proper nursing to curing the sick. Even when she describes the characteristics of her role model she uses this ability to cope with diarrhoea and sickness as an example. Her justification of the need for biology to understand 'conditions and medications' and her lack of understanding of the relevance of other disciplines suggest a student who finds tolerating ambiguity difficult.

In the nursery placement where she feels the only skill she has learned was cleaning paint pots suggests a very field-dependent approach to learning where the skill is not embedded in a wider set of behaviours or consideration of the environment. This reinforces Raskin's (1986) findings that field-dependent students tended to report careers in the helping areas.

Proper nurses work in hospital, concentrating on skills and tasks such as the Glasgow Coma Scale, giving out drugs and taking blood pressures:

> ... he did his job and the drugs and the paperwork and the things that you consider roles of the nurse *but* [researcher's emphasis] he would also spend time with the family and relatives talking to them or taking them out into the garden.

The 'but' in this sentence implies a definite difference between what the real job of nursing is and the social things that are on the periphery:

> ... he was like that because it was a relaxed atmosphere and I am sure he would have acted differently in a hospital.

Discussion

It would appear that Ha is a person with low self-esteem who has been attracted to nursing because of the gain in personal reward that results from caring (Barker et al., 1996; Yates & McDaniel, 1994). Her mention of the need for control lends itself to the nurse–patient relationship which has a power balance that enables her to maintain control at work that she may not have in her personal life. If she could be helped to overcome her problems and develop self-awareness, she could perhaps contribute to patient care with increased empathy (Kenny, 1994).

Ha could be the young girl mentioned in a recruitment commercial, wherein a young girl in a nurse's outfit with a bandaged teddy bear was captioned: 'The best nurses have the essential qualifications before they go to school' (Vousden, 1989: 25). In her dismissal of certain elements of her educational course, she is undermining relevance of wider issues necessary to prepare a nurse to promote health instead of care for sickness. Whilst she doesn't suggest that these are innate skills, she does suggest her socialisation played a key role in the person she is and she does expect to go on changing as she gets older.

There is evidence that she may be right about growing out of needing to please and taking more responsibility for herself as she gets older. Ha is currently in a very multiplicity phase of thinking (Perry, 1970), whereby she perceives diversity but interprets it as individuals have a right to their opinion, but she cannot understand it herself. In wanting clear boundaries, she also needs to know what authority wants to hear as the right answer. Relativistic thinking whereby the individual comes to understand that all knowledge is contextual is usually associated with moving into an internal locus of control. However, Ha's scores were only just above the median split putting her in this category. Analysis of the locus of control scores suggests that maturity may play a part in the change from external to internal as more students over the age or 25 had consistent internal locus of control and most of the students under the age of 25 had consistent external scores. There is also more ambivalence in the younger age group with more variation in the scores across the three years.

The inability to recognise boundaries is particularly worrying in the light of the recent UKCC publication on practitioner–client relationships and the prevention of abuse, (UKCC, 1999) paragraph eight states:

> Boundaries define the limits of behaviour, which allows a client and a practitioner to engage safely in a therapeutic caring relationship. These boundaries are based upon trust, respect and the appropriate use of power. The relationship between registered nurses ... and their clients is a therapeutic caring relationship, which must focus solely upon meeting the health or care needs of the client. It is not established to build personal or social contacts for practitioners. Moving the focus of care away from meeting the client's needs towards meeting the practitioner's own needs is an unacceptable abuse of power.

Barker et al. (1996) suggest that nurses who overcome their personal problems and develop self-awareness can contribute to patient care with increased empathy, but if they do not recognise, or cannot accept, the presence of their own vulnerability they might be sorely restricted in the practice of their art. This suggests that an important aspect of the educational programme should be developing self-awareness because it is unlikely that a shift is going to occur in the professional attitude of a person whose need for control and lack of awareness of boundaries is so pronounced.

On reflection the idea of the deviant case is quite compelling because it attempts to give credence to a view that does not fit in with the mainstream view and may shed some light on the 'other'. However, at the point in my journey where it would appear that my own story is deviant I am left with a puzzle. Perhaps there are no deviant cases, perhaps there are just lots more individual stories waiting to be told, stories that are sometimes difficult to tell, that need support and understanding in the telling. Without which it occurs to me nurses will go on perpetuating the myths of the good nurse, free of baggage on which the stereotype has too long rested. From which the real problems like Beverly Allitt (Clothier, 1994) emerge as some kind of pathologically needy person far removed from the norm rather than at just one end of a continuum of a variety of personal needs, which if not talked about will remain undetected. Just as I remain unconvinced about the philosophical pursuit of individualism in the Western world and can find very little evidence to suggest it is beneficial to the members of society it is purported to help, I remain sceptical about the objectivity of mainstream research. The deviant case may be a 'disconfirmation of the pattern' as Potter (1996: 138) says, but it may also be the plaintive voice of that silent minority of people whose voice is unheard.

Notes

* Celebrated author of many books including *Reflecting Men: At twice their natural size.*
(S. Cline & D. Spender, 1987.)

References

Barker, P., Reynolds, B., Whitehill, I. & Novak, V. (1996) 'Working with mental distress'. *Nursing Times*, **92** (2), 25–7.

Begley, C.M. (1996) 'Using triangulation in nursing research'. *Journal of Advanced Nursing*, **24**: 4, 122–8.

Benner, P. (1984) *From Novice to Expert – excellence and power in clinical nursing practice*. Menlo Park, CA: Addison Wesley.

Benner, P. & Tanner, C. (1987) 'How expert nurses use intuition'. *American Journal of Nursing*, **87** (1), 23–31.

Clarke, B., James, C. & Kelly, J. (1996) 'Reflective practice: reviewing the issues and refocusing the debate'. *International Journal of Nursing Studies*, **33** (2), 171–180.

Cline, S. & Spender, D. (1987) *Reflecting men: At twice their natural size*. London: Deutsch.

Clothier, C. (1994) *The Allitt Inquiry*, London: HMSO.

Flew, A. (1989) *A Dictionary of Philosophy*. 3rd edn. Basingstoke: Macmillan.

Guba, E.G. & Lincoln, Y.S. (1981) *Effective Evaluation*. San Francisco: Jossey Bass.

Jung, C.G. (1958) *The Undiscovered Self*. Massachusetts: Little, Brown.

Kelly, G.A. (1980) 'The psychology of optimal man', in Landfield, A.W. & Leitner, L.M. (eds) *Personal Construct Psychology: Psychotherapy and Personality*. London: John Wiley.

Kenny, C. (1994) 'Nursing Intuition: can it be researched?' *British Journal of Nursing*, **3** (22), 1191–5.

McCaugherty, D. (1991) 'The theory-practice gap in nurse education: its causes and possible solutions'. *Journal of Advanced Nursing*, **16**: 9, 1055–61.

Mead, G.H. (1934) *Mind, Self and Society*, Chicago: University of Chicago Press.

Meleis, A.I. (1991) *Theoretical Nursing: Development and Progress*. 2nd edn. Philadelphia: Lippincott.

Muncey, T. (2000) 'The Good Nurse: Born or Made? The implications for selection and retention from an investigation of the relative importance of previous socialisation and current education of nurses'. Unpublished PhD Thesis. Cranfield University.

Muncey, T. (1998) 'The pregnant adolescent: Sexually ignorant or destroyer of societies values?' in Morrissey, M. (ed.) (1998) *Sexuality and Healthcare: A Human Dilemma*. Salisbury: Mark Allen. Ch. 7.

Nolan, M. & Behi, R. (1995) 'Triangulation: the best of all worlds?' *British Journal of Nursing*, **14** (14), 829–32.

Perry, W.G. (1970) *Forms of Intellectual and Ethical Development in the College Years*. New York: Holt, Rinehart and Winston.

Potter, J. (1996) 'Discourse analysis and constructionist approaches: theoretical background' in Richardson, J.T.E. (ed.) *Handbook of Qualitative Research Methods for Psychology and the Social Sciences*. Leicester: BPS Books.

Raskin, E. (1986) 'Counselling implications of field-dependence in an educational setting', in Berttini, M. and Pizzamiglio, L. and Wapner, S. (eds) *Field Dependence in Psychological Theory, Research and Application*. New Jesey: Erlbaum Hillsdale.

Redfern, S.J. & Norman, I.J. (1994) 'Validity through triangulation'. *Nurse Researcher*, **2** (2), 41–56.

Rew, L. (1989) 'Childhood sexual exploitation: long term effects among a group of nursing students'. *Issues in Mental Health Nursing*, **10**: 2, 181–91.

UKCC (1999) *Practitioner–Client Relationships and the Prevention of Abuse*. London: UKCC.

Vousden, M. (1989) 'Selling Nurses'. *Nursing Times*, **85** (34), 25–9.

Wetherell, M. (1989) 'Linguistic Repertoires and Literary criticism: New Directions for a Social Psychology of Gender' in Holloway, W. *Subjectivity and Method in Psychology*. London: Sage. Ch. 5.

Yates, J.G. & McDaniel, J.L. (1994) 'Are you losing yourself in co-dependency?' *American Journal of Nursing*, April, 32–6.

10 Reflexive Research and the Therapeutic Use of Self

Gary Rolfe

This final chapter explores the issues surrounding the use of self in the research process. In addressing these issues, I am aware of the problems of definition and conceptualisation of self, particularly in constructionist and postmodern discourses. However, these issues have been discussed elsewhere in this book, and whilst I am sympathetic to the view that self is co-constructed during the encounter with other, and even to the postmodern assertion that self-presence is impossible, I am concerned here with pragmatics rather than with metaphysics. For the purpose of this chapter, then, I will take what might be termed the common-sense view that self has a more or less stable meaning and that it is to some extent possible to know both the self of others (intersubjectivity) and my own self (self-presence).

As we shall see, the concern of most traditional approaches to research (if, indeed, they are concerned with it at all) is with how to eliminate self from the research setting; how, as one writer has put it, to depopulate the research text. If the aim of research is to produce general knowledge and theories about the world at large, then this concern is understandable, since we would not wish our theory of everything to be contaminated by the particular. However, nursing research, or at least *clinical* nursing research, should be concerned with nursing practice, and nursing practice is a series of *individual encounters* between individual people. In this case, general knowledge and theory is of little practical use; what we need is knowledge about people rather than about populations.

My concern in this chapter is therefore with ways of putting self back into the research process, with repopulating research texts. This concern begins where most other research texts end; that is, with the notion of using self as a research tool, a phrase that has now become so over used in qualitative research texts that it is almost a cliché. From there, I explore the feminist notion of the *therapeutic* use of self in research, and then move onwards and outwards to the idea of self as a tool to explore *itself*, that is, with *reflective* research. Finally, I attempt to close the circle by examining how this self-knowledge can be applied back into practice in the form of *reflexive* research, that is, how introspective knowledge about self can lead directly to changes in the outside world. I begin, however, with the traditional positivist approach to dealing with the self of both the researcher and the researched.

Research and the suppression of self

The aim of nursing research is usually described as the production of generalisable knowledge; that is, of knowledge that applies beyond the research subjects from whom it was obtained. This general aim is explicitly stated in almost all definitions of nursing research, and has been formalised in statements made by a number of authoritative and governing bodies such as the Department of Health in the UK, which has defined nursing research as rigorous and systematic enquiry 'designed to lead to generalisable contributions to knowledge' (DoH, 1993: 6). Such definitions have certain implications, or indeed, imperatives for the ways in which data are collected and presented as part of the research process. Most importantly for the purposes of this chapter, if the findings of the study are to be extended beyond the sample from which the data were collected, then that sample must be presented as representative of a wider population. In other words, each person in the research sample represents not herself, but a particular social, demographic or other group, and so the researcher is not interested in what the data collected from any individual says about the subject as a person, but rather what it says about people in general. Research subjects are therefore not valued as individual people for their individual traits, but only to the extent that their individuality is representative of some greater collective whole. As Benney and Hughes pointed out concerning research interviews:

> As an encounter between these two particular people the typical interview has no meaning; it is conceived in a framework of other, comparable meetings between other couples, each recorded in such fashion that elements of communication in common can be easily isolated from more idiosyncratic qualities. (1970: 197)

Typically, then, the generalisability or external validity of the study is maximised by suppressing the individuality of the research subjects and, in effect, presenting them as research *objects,* as decontextualised examples or representatives of some greater whole. In the terminology of Martin Buber (1958), the relationship between researcher and researched is one of I–it rather than I–thou. More specifically, the researcher presents as what Buber referred to as a demoniac thou who is recognised by her research subjects as thou, as a person, but who perceives them merely as it, as objects.

However, it is not only the individual traits of these research objects that can threaten the generalisabilty of the study, but also those of the researcher herself. The researcher must therefore convince her readers that her particular and unique attitudes, beliefs, prejudices and so on, exerted no influence over the design, execution or presentation of the study. There are two ways in which the researcher might tackle this problem. Firstly, she can attempt to present herself as identical in all respects to all other researchers, indeed, to all other people; in other words, to convince her readers that it would make no difference *who* conducted the study. Secondly, she can remove herself from the scene of the research entirely and present the study as if it somehow designed, conducted and wrote up itself.

The first strategy is usually aided by the sleight of hand of writing up the findings in the third person. To write that 'I administered a questionnaire' is to suggest that a particular individual with particular and unique views and biases became subjectively entangled in the data collection process. On the other hand, to write that the researcher administered the questionnaire is to suggest a Platonic ideal, a disembodied and perfect researching machine, devoid of individual quirks; or, at least, that if she (it?) does have individual quirks, they are generic quirks, matched and therefore cancelled out by those of that very same researcher (or of a perfect copy of that researcher), *the* researcher, who appears to have written almost every other published study.

The second strategy of disappearing from the scene of the research is usually achieved by writing in the passive case. No longer do we read that the researcher administered the questionnaire, but simply that the questionnaire *was adminis-tered*. As Michael Billig observed, 'much social science is *depopulated*, filled with abstract concepts, broad judgements and descriptions of general processes, but it is devoid of people' (1994: 151). The main players in the act of research have all left the stage; the depopulation of the text, and with it, all possibility of individual bias, is complete. In either case, the researcher not only has an I–it relationship with her research objects, but also with herself. In presenting herself as an objective researcher, she presents herself also as merely an object.

We can see, then, that if the purpose of research is to make large-scale statisti-cal generalisations from a relatively small sample to a wider population, then the relationship that the researcher has with those whom she is researching, and also with herself, is compromised to the extent that it disappears completely; objects might interact with one another, but they do not form relationships. The idea of the research process offering the possibility of any sort of relationship, therapeu-tic or otherwise, is therefore not only discouraged by the positivist paradigm, but is completely written out as unwarranted and inconceivable.

However, although this detached positivist approach continues to be promoted as the dominant research paradigm in nursing, it is by no means the *only* para-digm, and a number of alternatives espouse aims other than the production of generalisable knowledge. In particular, we might identify three alternative aims of antipositivist research:

- the production of knowledge about the individual subject or clearly defined small groups of subjects on/with whom the research is conducted;
- the production of knowledge about the researcher herself; and
- direct improvements to practice brought about by the research act itself.

The first of these aims is most readily met using a case study or ethnographic methodology, the second aim calls for a more reflective methodology, and the final aim implies some form of action research intervention. All, however, sug-gest an ideographic focus to the research; that is, they involve intensive study of unique phenomena in particular cases rather than wide-ranging studies that seek to discover general laws. Clearly, then, the imperative in ideographic research is not to write the researcher and the researched *out* of the study, but rather to write them *in*. Once we open up the possibility of the world of research being inhabited by living, breathing people, each with their own individual traits and differences, then research becomes a series of encounters between different (and, we might add, constantly changing) selves. In other words, ideographic research is consti-tuted by a series of ongoing I–thou relationships, constantly formulated and reformulated, either serendipitously or as part of a deliberate research strategy.

The many different ways in which these selves can and do interact and interrelate in the production of ideographic knowledge about the research subject is the focus of the next part of this chapter.

Research and the use of self

Most researchers who work within an ideographic paradigm would, to some extent, subscribe to the idea of the self (whatever they take that to mean) as a research tool with which to explore the world of the research subject. However, certain methodologies attribute more value to this particular tool than do others, and these differences of emphasis are apparent even *within* methodologies. For example, Heideggarian or hermeneutic phenomenologists encourage the creative use of the lifeworld of the researcher in understanding the lifeworld of the researched, whereas phenomenologists from the Husserlian tradition advocate bracketing as a way of minimising the impact of the researchers lifeworld. Furthermore, the exact shape of the tool depends to some extent on the stage of the study at which the self is to be deployed. For example, the tool of self might be employed during an interview to put the research subject at her ease and to build a trusting relationship in order to maximise both the quality and quantity of the data. In contrast, self might be employed during data analysis as a way of bringing the experience of the researcher to the interpretation of the data. In either case, the deployment of self as a research tool is based on the assumption that human knowledge is literally constructed during inquiry and hence is 'inevitably entwined with the perceptual frames, histories, and values of the inquirer' (Greene 1998: 390). We have seen, then, that most ideographic researchers regard an I–thou relationship with their research subjects as an essential aspect of the research process.

However, some writers have critiqued this relationship as not being truly authentic, indeed, as not really meeting the criteria of a relationship at all. For example, Michelle Fine has argued how the hyphen that connects Self–Other (that is, researcher and researched) at once 'separates and merges personal identities with our inventions of others' (Fine, 1998: 131). Thus, even qualitative researchers:

> ... self-consciously carry no voice, body, race, class, or gender and no interests into their texts. Narrators seek to shelter themselves in the text, as if they were transparent. They recognise no hyphen. (1998: 138)

This is the converse of the I–it problem, where the relationship between researcher and researched is not objectified but subjectified. The relationship falls apart not through too much distance, but because there is no distance at all, no hyphen. As Buber maintained, the meaning of the I–thou relationship is not so much in the coming together of two people, but in the space between them, that is, in the hyphen itself. Without the hyphen, there can be no relationship.

A rather different critique of the authenticity of the research relationship comes from feminist researchers such as Ann Oakley (1981), who points out that true

I–thou relationships have to be reciprocal; that both parties should enter into them with the expectation of both giving *and* receiving (although, as we have seen, there exists the possibility of the one-sided demoniac thou relationship). When the researcher uses her self as a therapeutic tool, it is fairly apparent what she is receiving *from* (and perhaps also what she is giving *to*) the relationship, but it is less clear just what exactly the research subject is getting, apart from the warm glow of giving without expecting anything in return. From the standpoint of feminist methodology, then, there is an imperative for the researcher to give something back to the relationship, since as Oakley tells us 'there is no intimacy without reciprocity'. (1981: 49)

Oakley (1981) identified a number of ways in which the researcher can overtly offer something to the research subject in return for her time, effort and (as Oakley tells us) numerous cups of tea and the occasional meal. Firstly, she can openly and honestly answer requests for personal information such as 'What sort of person was I' and 'How did I come to be interested in this subject?' Secondly, she can offer advice on the issues that she is researching. This, as Oakley pointed out, directly contravenes the norms of social research which require a detached and even aloof stance on the part of the researcher, who is there to obtain information and to focus on the respondent, not himself (Goode & Hatt, 1952). However, as she noted of her own research into childbirth:

> The dilemma of a feminist interviewer interviewing women could be summarised by considering the practical application of some of the strategies recommended in the textbooks for meeting interviewee's questions. For example, these advise that such questions as, Which hole does the baby come out of? Does an epidural ever paralyse women? and Why is it dangerous to leave a small baby alone in the house? [all questions that Oakley had been asked during the course of her research] should be met with such responses from the interviewer as, I guess I haven't thought enough about it to give a good answer right now, or a head shaking gesture which suggests that's a hard one [quoted by Oakley from Goode & Hatt, 1952]. Also recommended is laughing off the request with the remark that my job at the moment is to get opinions, not to have them [quoted by Oakley from Selltiz et al., 1965]. (Oakley, 1981: 48)

For Oakley, such responses clearly will not do.

Thirdly, the researcher can offer friendship. Oakley tells us of her study on childbirth that:

> ... four years after the final interview I am still in touch with more than a third of the women I interviewed. Four have become close friends, several others I visit occasionally, and the rest write or telephone when they have something salient to report such as the birth of another child. (Oakley, 1981: 46)

And fourthly, she can offer help of a more practical kind:

> For instance, if the interview clashed with the demands of housework and motherhood I offered to, and often did, help with the work that had to be done. (Oakley, 1981: 47)

As Oakley is at pains to point out, this reciprocity is both uncommon in research relationships and is usually rejected as unscientific in its introduction of bias into the research setting. It therefore calls for a new conception of the research process in which bias is accepted as a naturally occurring phenomenon in *all* human inter-actions, including those necessitated in *all* social research paradigms, including positivism. Furthermore, reciprocity is not simply an issue of authenticity and feminist praxis. Oakley's study involved multiple interviews with the same women, and as she pointed out, without feeling that the interviewing process offered some personal satisfaction to them, interviewees would not be prepared to continue after the first interview (Oakley, 1981: 49).

We should not assume, however, that research relationships have to be *overtly* reciprocal as Oakley described in order to be authentic. We know from the vast body of literature on counselling, and particularly on non-directive and humanis-tic counselling (Rogers, 1974 for example), that in the right psychological condi-tions, simply being listened to whilst she tells her story can give something of value back to the research subject. It has to be stressed, however, that the condi-tions must be right and that there must be a commitment on the part of the researcher not simply to drop the relationship once it has met her need for research data. Thus, under certain conditions, what Oakley termed the 'therapeu-tic listener' role of the researcher can, of itself, offer a rich and rewarding relationship for both researcher and researched.

Clearly, the opposite is also true. If telling our story for the purpose of research can, at the same time, constitute a therapeutic relationship, then the therapy session can also form a site for research. This is perhaps best exemplified in the writing of Freud, where cases were written up and presented as research evidence for the emerging science (as Freud would have it) of psychoanalysis. As he pointed out in the *Prefatory Remarks* to his case study of Dora:

> … in my opinion the physician has taken upon himself duties not only towards the indi-vidual patient but towards science as well; and his duties towards science mean ulti-mately nothing else than his duties towards the many other patients who are suffering or will some day suffer from the same disorder. Thus it becomes the physician's duty to publish what he believes he knows of the causes and structure of hysteria … (Freud, 1977: 36)

Freud clearly regarded psychoanalysis not only as a method of therapy, but also as a form of research, and as Richards pointed out in their introduction to Freud's *Studies on Hysteria*, perhaps the most important of Freud's achievements was 'his invention of the first instrument for the scientific examination of the human mind' (1974: 35).

When we talk of the researcher using herself as the research tool, we therefore imply far more than simply bringing her own experience to the analysis of data, or even of using her skills as an interviewer to facilitate the smooth and accurate collection of valid data. If we subscribe to the idea of the authentic I–thou research interview, then the researcher must give something back to the research subject in the form of commitment, attention, respect and empathy. And, as Carl Rogers (1974) tells us, under these conditions the focus of the relationship, whatever its stated intentions, transcends the collection of data to become a therapeutic encounter in its own right.

Research and the exploration of self

I have, up to now, taken a fairly traditional view of ideographic research as the study of individual cases and small groups, and I have discussed some ways in which the researcher might use her self in her relationships with her research subjects (and, indeed, the extent to which she might view them as subjects rather than objects of her research). However, I argued earlier that the production of knowledge about others is only one of several aims or purposes of ideographic research, and I now wish to move beyond the traditional confines of the dyadic research relationship to explore the idea of research as a process of self-discovery; that is, the idea of researching my *own* self.

In one sense, the idea of the researcher exploring her own self in the research process is now well established, particularly in the case of doctoral students, who are often required to keep a reflective research journal. The aim of this journal is firstly to chart the progress of the study, but secondly and more importantly, to provide a space for the student to reflect on her own practice of research and in a sense to know herself as a researcher. However, this reflective approach to research is limited in the extent to which the researcher can fully come to know herself. If she wishes to explore aspects of her self other than that of her role as researcher, the study of self must become the *focus* of the research rather than simply part of the *process*. In other words, the focus of the study must be turned from the outer to the inner, from the thoughts, feelings, beliefs, attitudes and practices of the thou to those of the I, that is, of the researcher herself. Under these conditions, the researcher and the researched become one and the same person.

This introspective approach to doing research on oneself has a long history in philosophy that can be traced back to the inscription 'Know Thyself' on the doorway to the Greek temple of Delphi, and to Socrates' claim that the unexamined life is not worth living. However, it was first proposed as a social research method by Clark Moustakas (1961) and later developed by action researchers, ethnographers and phenomenologists.

For Moustakas (1990), true understanding of any phenomenon can only come about through a deep and personal engagement with that phenomenon in a process he referred to as 'heuristic research'. Thus:

> From the beginning and throughout an investigation, heuristic research involves self-search, self-dialogue, and self-discovery; the research question and the methodology flow out of inner awareness, meaning and inspiration. When I consider an issue, problem, or question, I enter into it fully. I focus on it with unwavering attention and interest. I search introspectively, meditatively, and reflectively into its nature and meaning. My primary task is to recognize whatever exists in my consciousness as a fundamental awareness, to receive and accept it, and then to dwell on its nature and possible meanings. With full and unqualified interest, I am determined to extend my understanding and knowledge of an experience. I begin the heuristic investigation with my own self-awareness and explicate that awareness with reference to a question or problem until an essential insight is achieved, one that will throw a beginning light onto a critical human experience. (Moustakas, 1990: 11)

In his original study into loneliness, Moustakas (1961) began with his own experience of contemplating life without his sick daughter and supplemented this self-dialogue with observations, interviews, biography and literature. However, even when turning to sources outside of self, the self of the researcher remained central to the research process. Thus, the interviews and observations undertaken by Moustakas were far removed from the classic form of scientific data collection, and pushed Oakley's dictum of no intimacy without reciprocity to its limits. In describing how he initiated his study in the hospital in which his daughter was being treated, Moustakas tells us that:

> Initially, I studied loneliness in its essential forms by putting myself into an open, ready state, into the lonely experiences of hospitalized children, and letting these experiences become the focus of my world. I listened. I watched. I stood by. In dialogue with the children, I tried to put into words the depth of their feelings. Sometimes my words touched a child and tears began to flow; sometimes the child formed words in response to my presence, and broke through the numbness and the dehumanising impact of the hospital atmosphere and practice. In a strong sense, loneliness became my existence. (1990: 95)

Perhaps we should just stop and ponder for a moment on the probable reaction of a modern-day ethical committee to a proposal for a research study which 'had no design or purpose, no object or end, and no hypotheses or assumptions' (Moustakas, 1981: 208), where the methodology is to listen, to watch, to stand by, and ultimately to let loneliness become my existence, and where part of the process involved reducing children to tears. And yet Moustakas clearly sees reducing children to tears as not only ethically sound, but almost as an ethical imperative, intended to break through 'the numbness and the dehumanising impact of the hospital atmosphere and practice'. And so we return to the inescapable conclusion that research, when conducted in a certain way, is also a therapeutic encounter either with 'I' or with 'thou'. As O'Hara tells us, 'This view acknowledges healing as a *natural consequence* of a successful moment in a progressive search for truth' (O'Hara, 1986: 177).

As you might imagine, this self-conscious (we might almost say self-centred) approach to research is not without its detractors. We have already anticipated some of the possible ethical objections to such an unstructured and overtly therapeutic methodology (or perhaps we should say non-methodology), and no doubt researchers from a more positivist tradition would critique it for being almost totally lacking in validity. Certainly, if we assess validity in traditional terms as the extent to which a study conforms to certain methodological rules and guidelines, then such criticism is undoubtedly warranted. But consider this: Moustakas claimed that 'since the publication of *Loneliness,* I have received approximately 2000 letters that validate my portrayal of the nature of loneliness in modern life' (1990: 97). If, as many qualitative researchers tell us, judgements about the validity or truthfulness of a study lie not with the academic researcher but with the reader and potential user of the findings, then Moustakas' work has achieved an almost unprecedented validity check beyond the imaginings and expectations of most researchers.

A more fundamental objection comes not from researchers but from philosophers, who consider such an extreme form of self-reflexivity to be unattainable. How, they ask, is it possible for consciousness to employ consciousness in order to study consciousness; or more simply, how can the self observe itself? Max van Manen (1997) has pointed out that the very process of reflecting on my consciousness serves to alter the state that I am attempting to reflect on. Perhaps I am angry, and wish to learn more about my anger by reflecting on it. As van Manen observed, as soon as I begin to reflect on my anger I am no longer angry but, rather, inquisitive or attentive. As the *Oxford Dictionary of Philosophy* dryly notes in its entry for 'self': '**Self** – The elusive 'I' that shows an alarming tendency to disappear when we try to introspect it' (Blackburn, 1994: 344).

Moustakas deals with this objection by separating out the research process into a number of phases. Thus, the second phase following the initial engagement with the research question is 'immersion', during which 'the researcher lives the question in waking, sleeping, and even dream states' (1990: 28). Then comes 'incubation', when the researcher retreats from the intense, concentrated focus of the question (1990: 28). However, although the researcher is no longer 'living the question', or indeed even consciously thinking about it, 'the period of incubation allows the inner workings of the tacit dimension and intuition to continue to clarify and extend understanding on levels outside the immediate awareness' (1990: 29). This is followed by 'illumination', a 'breakthrough into conscious awareness' (1990: 29) of the incubated ideas, which can now be explicated and synthesised into the finished report that might be presented as a narrative, poem, story, drawing, painting or some other creative form. To return to the earlier example of anger, the insights come not in the immersion phase when the researcher is actually living her anger, but in the incubation and illumination phases when the experiences of anger are being processed unconsciously and surfaced back into awareness.

Other methodologies later applied the more or less >pure= introspection of heuristic research to their own particular ends. For example, hermeneutic phenomenologists such as Hans-Georg Gadamer regard research into our own selves and our prejudices (pre-judgements) as a precursor and prerequisite to understanding and interpreting the selves of others. Thus 'our prejudices do not constitute a wilful blindness which prevents us grasping the truth; rather they are a platform from which we launch our very attempt at understanding' (Moran, 2000: 278). For hermeneutic phenomenologists, then, introspection becomes an interpretive tool.

Over the past ten years, ethnographers have also attempted to apply the introspective heuristic method to their own ends. This 'autoethnography' has been described by Denzin as 'a turning of the ethnographic gaze inward on the self (auto), while maintaining the outward gaze of ethnography, looking at the larger context wherein self experiences occur' (Denzin, 1997: 227). Autoethnography usually takes the form of written narrative accounts of events from the researcher's own life, often presented in a literary or poetic style (see, for example, Ellis & Bochner, 1996). However, these texts are first and foremost ethnographies and must therefore do more than simply 'put the self of the writer on the line or tell realist, emotional stories about self-renewal, crisis, and catharsis' (Denzin, 1997: 200). Rather, 'the tale being told should reflect back on, be entangled in, and critique this current historical moment and its discontents' (1997: 200). The aim of autoethnography is therefore to employ self as a tool to explore the wider culture in which the researcher participates.

Similarly, some action researchers such as John Elliott and Jean McNiff have emphasised the importance of self-reflection as a means of challenging and transforming practice. This approach to action research has been described as:

> ... the systematic study of attempts to change and improve ... practice by groups of participants by means of their own practical actions and by means of their own reflection upon the effects of those actions. (Ebbutt, 1985: 156)

Taken to its logical conclusion, this approach results in what John Heron (1981) has called 'co-operative inquiry', in which the barriers between the researchers and the researched are completely dissolved and the co-inquirers are engaged in a deep and sustained investigation of themselves and each other.

In all of the above examples, the aim of the reflective process is to provide knowledge about the self of the researcher, which is then used to further the aims of the research in one way or another. I have referred to this reflective approach as Level 3 research, in contrast to Level 1 positivist research and Level 2 interpretative research. Thus:

> Level 3 or reflective research is concerned primarily with researching one's own practice. It is an individual endeavour whose aim is to generate personal knowledge and informal theory from a retrospective, systematic and detailed analysis of what happened in the practice setting. (Rolfe, 1996: 61–2)

Level 3 research is particularly appropriate to practice disciplines such as nursing, since it provides an alternative to the dominant technical rationality model. Technical rationality, which has become the 'gold standard' paradigm of nursing research, proposes that knowledge and theory should be generated *for* practice by professional researchers through a process of looking in objectively on practice from the outside. In contrast, Level 3 research suggests that knowledge and theory for practice might be generated *from* practice by practitioners themselves through a process of looking subjectively at practice from the inside.

One of the consequences of technical rationality that reflective research attempts to address is the problem of the theory–practice gap. Under the technical rationality paradigm, research and practice are separate activities undertaken by different people, and so a gap is created at the point of implementation where the research finding is handed over from researcher to practitioner. In contrast, reflective research is usually conducted by the practitioner herself into her own practice. Thus:

> Reflective research therefore eliminates the theory–practice gap by ensuring that theory developed out of clinical encounters with a particular patient is directly applied back into the nurse's practice with that same patient. (Rolfe, 1996: 62)

However, this reflective model clearly has political consequences in the way that it more or less writes the professional researcher out of the research process, and we should therefore not be surprised to see a concerted effort on the part of the dominant paradigm to negate or discredit reflective practitioner-based research.

One way of putting reflective research in its place is by labelling it as soft in relation to the hard science of technical rationality. Thus, positivist researchers describe themselves as being hard in the sense of being tough, rigorous and unbending, whereas practitioner-researchers are considered soft because they are, by implication, weak, lacking in rigour and easily swayed. Many researchers regard these labels simply as neutral, value-free descriptions of the two paradigms, and even qualitative researchers describe themselves as soft without too much thought about the origin and implication of the term. However, Pauline Bart has observed that this dichotomy is actually based on a very male-oriented metaphor that privileges the hard at the expense of the soft:

> We speak of hard data as being better than soft data, hard science better than soft science, hard money better than soft money. In the fifties, one was criticised for being soft on communism. This is of course a male sexual metaphor, so since discovering this, I have substituted a metaphor based on female sexual experience and refer to wet and dry data. (Bart, 1974: 1)

By resisting and reversing the male metaphor, Bart has also resisted and (to some extent) reversed the hierarchical value system that it implies. Furthermore, her alternative terminology is, in fact, far more appropriate as a description of the technical rationality and the reflective paradigms. The technical rational researcher is dry and objective; she refuses to get excited, to become aroused by her encounters with the subjects of her research, whom she views as objects and means to an end. In contrast, the reflective researcher is passionately immersed and involved both in the topic and in the process of the research to the point of entanglement. The wet practitioner-researcher is therefore unable and unwilling to distinguish between her two roles.

Shifting the metaphor only slightly, Donald Schön has observed that:

> In the varied topography of professional practice, there is a high, hard ground overlooking a swamp. On the high ground, manageable problems lend themselves to solution through the application of research-based theory and technique. In the swampy lowland, messy, confusing problems defy technical solution. (Schön 1987: 3)

For Schön, the high, hard ground overlooking a swamp is the dry land of detached and objective technical rationality, whereas the swampy lowland, [where] messy, confusing problems defy technical solution is the wetlands of engaged and subjective practice. Furthermore, the solutions to the messy, confusing problems of practice lie not in technical rationality, where the researcher does her best to keep her feet on dry land, but in reflection-on-action, which attempts to draw out the knowledge and theory that resides in practice itself. This knowledge and theory is accessible only to the researcher who is also a practising nurse, and so for Schön, the researcher has no choice but to descend into the swamp.

Research and the immersion of self

The descent of the researcher into the swampy lowlands is only the first stage in a process that fully integrates the researcher with the practitioner. The practitioner who reflects on her own practice might be both a researcher and a practitioner, but the two roles are sequential and cyclical. First she practices, then she reflects on her practice, then she applies what she has learnt back into her practice, and so on in a reflective spiral. Practice is likely to improve as a result of this reflection-on-action, but the basic aim is to generate knowledge, albeit a rather different kind of knowledge from that produced through dry positivist research.

As we saw earlier, however, the third aim of ideographic research is directly to improve practice through the research act itself, and this suggests a far more intimate link between research and practice. For Schön, this full and final integration between research and practice is achieved through the process of reflection-*in*-action, in which reflection takes place *in situ,* in the midst of practice. Thus:

> ... phrases like 'thinking on your feet', 'keeping your wits about you', and 'learning by doing' suggest not only that we can think about doing but that we can think about doing something while doing it. (1983: 54)

When the practitioner reflects *in* rather than *on* practice, the roles of researcher and practitioner are finally merged. As Schön tells us, 'when someone reflects-in-action, *he becomes a researcher in the practice context.* He is not dependent on the categories of established theory and technique, but constructs a new theory of the unique case' (1983: 68, my emphasis). I refer to this form of practice-based research as Level 4 research or reflexive research, in which 'theory is tested by modifying practice, but practice also changes theory in a virtuous circle. Theory and practice are therefore developing in direct response to one another in a process that can continue indefinitely' (Rolfe, 1996: 38).

It is this integration of thinking and acting that prompted Schön (1983) to refer to reflection-in-action also as on-the-spot experimenting, and he identified three ways in which it might take place. Firstly, on-the-spot experimenting can be a simple, pre-scientific form of trial and error that he referred to as 'exploratory experimentation'. Secondly, it can be an action that is carried out in order to produce an *intended* change, which he referred to as 'move testing'. Thirdly, and most importantly, it can be a form of hypothesis testing in which the practitioner formulates a theory about the clinical situation she is faced with, derives a hypothesis from that theory, and tests her hypothesis by acting on the situation. This process bears a strong resemblance to Popper's hypothetico-deductivist method of scientific research, and as Schön pointed out:

> If, for a given hypothesis, its predicted consequences fit what is observed, and the predictions derived from alternative hypotheses conflict with observation, then we can say that the first hypothesis has been *confirmed* and the others, *disconfirmed.* (1983: 146, his emphasis)

The reflexive practitioner who reflects in action is therefore engaged in a constant dialogue with herself as she formulates theories, tests hypotheses and adjusts her practice accordingly. Her practice is a form of research in which '[s]he carries out an experiment which serves to generate both a new understanding of the phenomena and a change in the situation' (Schön 1983: 68).

However, if reflection-in-action claims to be a form of scientific research, then it has an obligation to respond to questions about its validity. Clearly, the positivist idea of validity as a recourse to some kind of objective benchmark of the research construct is completely outside the remit of reflexive research. However, in any practice-based discipline, the *ultimate* measure of validity has to be the extent to which the research study improves practice. According to this standard, the validity of positivist research can only be measured if or when the findings are eventually applied in the practice setting, and it is of little consequence that the study measured what it claimed to measure if it does not contribute to better practice. But of course this is the strength of reflexive research, since the practitioner-researcher receives continuous feedback about the effectiveness of her interventions and the research continues until it *does* make a positive change to practice. If reflection-in-action is seen as a continuous process of testing out hypotheses and modifying practice accordingly, then it has a very effective validity check built into it.

However, reflection-in-action is not simply the process of theorising and experimenting in practice. As Schön points out, it also has a second component:

> … both ordinary people and professional practitioners often think about what they are doing, sometimes even while doing it. Stimulated by surprise, *they turn thought back* on action and *on the knowing which is implicit in action.* They may ask themselves, for example, 'What features do I notice when I recognise this thing? What are the criteria by which I make this judgement? What procedures am I enacting when I perform this skill? How am I framing the problem that I am trying to solve?'. (Schön 1983: 50, my emphasis)

Thus, as well as turning of thought back on action through hypothesising, thought is also turned back on the knowing which is implicit in action. The reflexive practitioner-researcher is reflecting not only on her practice in a process of on-the-spot experimenting, but is simultaneously reflecting on that very *process* of her on-the-spot experimenting, a sort of reflection about reflection or meta-reflection that resembles Casement's (1985) internal supervisor.

This meta-reflection adds an education component to those of practice and research. Clearly, the practitioner-researcher is able to think critically about her practice *on the spot,* as it is happening. She is therefore *learning* not only about her patients but also about her self, and is in a position to implement this learning directly back into practice. But more importantly, she is learning not just about the content of her practice but also about the process, that is, about *how* she practices. This knowledge is of particular importance to the advanced or autonomous practitioner for three important reasons. Firstly, it enables her to begin to understand the principles and processes that underpin her *modus operandi* in ways that are simply not available to most practitioners. She is, in effect, able to gain access to the tacit knowledge that practitioners usually attribute to gut feeling or intuition.

Secondly, she is able to offer justification for her practice in a far more articulate way than the usual 'I just knew the right things to say and do, but don't ask me how I knew them' or 'I just knew intuitively'. This is important not only as *evidence* for practice, but also as a way of closing the theory-practice gap. As Schön tells us:

> When people use terms such as 'art' and 'intuition', they usually intend to terminate discussion rather than to open up inquiry. It is as though the practitioner says to his academic colleague, 'While I do not accept your view of knowledge, I cannot describe my own'. Sometimes, indeed, the practitioner appears to say 'My kind of knowledge is indescribable, or even I will not attempt to describe it lest I paralyse myself'. These attitudes have contributed to a widening rift between the universities and the professions, research and practice, thought and action. (Schön, 1983: viii)

By beginning to describe the knowledge on which her practice is constructed, the reflexive practitioner-researcher is able to go some way towards closing this rift between research and practice.

And thirdly, the reflexive practitioner-researcher is able to share this knowledge with colleagues and students. Thus, she is educating not just herself as she practices, but also everyone around her, including her patients. This is clearly in keeping with the latest developments in the role of the nurse consultant, in celebrating and rewarding the expertise of clinicians rather than moving them sideways into managerial or academic roles. Writing several years before the concept of the nurse consultant I argued:

> The most significant consequence of this shift in importance from research-based knowledge to experiential knowledge and praxis is that the status of nursing practice and the ward-based, clinical nurse is elevated in accordance with her new role as researcher and generator of theory. She no longer merely applies theories dictated by educationalists and researchers; she is an educationalist and a researcher. (Rolfe, 1996: 43)

Conclusion

By excluding the idea of self from the research process, the roles of researcher, practitioner and educationalist are kept irretrievably separate. In this technical rationality model, the job of the researcher is to generate abstract, decontextualised and depopulated knowledge; the job of the educator is to disseminate it; and the job of the practitioner is to apply it by recontextualising and repopulating it. This chapter has explored a variety of attempts by researchers and practitioners to reintroduce the self of the research subject and, more importantly, the researcher, back into the research process. This repopulation culminated in a discussion of the reflexive practitioner-researcher-educator, for whom reflection-in-action provides an integrative methodology for combining the three roles and raising the profile and status of the clinical nurse. Reflection-in-action is not only a form of reflexive research in which improvement to practice takes place as part of the research process itself, but it also involves reflecting on the research process as it is occurring. Thus, the self becomes fully immersed in the research process: it is at once the researcher, the researched, the topic of the research, the research tool and the research supervisor. And yet, despite this introspective, almost solipsistic focus, the result is eminently practical, far more so, in fact, than most traditional forms of social research. For the outcome of reflexive research of this kind is not only new knowledge and theories about practice, but an actual improvement in practice (albeit on a micro, individual level) that is rarely achieved through technical rationality and evidence-based practice. The promise, indeed the irony, of researching our self is that it has the potential to make the world a better place.

References

Bart, P. (1974) 'Male views of female sexuality, from Freud's phallacies to Fisher's inexact test'. Paper presented at the second national meeting, special section on Psychosomatic Obstetrics and Gynaecology, Florida: Key Biscayne.

Benney, M. & Hughes, E.C. (1970) 'Of sociology and the interview' in Denzin, N.K. (ed.) *Sociological Methods: A Source Book.* London: Butterworth.

Billig, M. (1994) 'Sod Baudrillard! Or ideology critique in Disney World' in Simons, H.W. & Billig, M. (eds) *After Postmodernism: Reconstructing Ideology Critique.* London: Sage.

Blackburn, S. (1994) *The Oxford Dictionary of Philosophy.* Oxford: OUP.

Buber, M. (1958) *I and Thou.* Edinburgh: T&T Clark.

Casement, P. (1985) *On Learning from the Patient.* London: Routledge.

Denzin, N. (1997) *Interpretive Ethnography.* Thousand Oaks: Sage.

Department of Health (1993) *Report of the Taskforce on the Strategy for Research in Nursing, Midwifery and Health Visiting.* London: HMSO.

Ebbutt, D. (1985) 'Educational action research: some general concerns and specific quibbles' in Burgess, R.G. (ed.) *Issues in Educational Research: Qualitative Methods.* Lewes: Falmer Press.

Ellis, C. & Bochner, A.P. (eds) (1996) *Composing Ethnography: Alternative Forms of Qualitative Writing.* London: Sage.

Fine, M. (1998) 'Working the hyphens: reinventing "self" and "other" in qualitative research' in Denzin, N.K. & Lincoln, Y.S. (eds) *The Landscape of Qualitative Research.* Thousand Oaks: Sage.

Freud, S. (1977) *Case Histories I: 'Dora' and 'Little Hans'.* Harmondsworth: Penguin.

Goode, W.J. & Hatt, P.K. (1952) *Methods in Social Research.* New York: McGraw Hill.

Greene, J.C. (1998) 'Qualitative program evaluation: practice and promise' in Denzin, N.K. & Lincoln, Y.S. (eds) *Collecting and Interpreting Qualitative Materials.* Thousand Oaks: Sage.

Heron, J. (1981) 'Philosophical basis for a new paradigm' in Reason, P. & Rowan, J. (eds) *Human Inquiry: A Sourcebook of New Paradigm Research.* Chichester: John Wiley.

Moran, D. (2000) *Introduction to Phenomenology.* London: Routledge.

Moustakas, C. (1961) *Loneliness.* Englewood Cliffs: Prentice Hall.

Moustakas, C. (1981) *Rhythms, Rituals and Relationships.* Detroit: Center for Humanistic Studies.

Moustakas, C. (1990) *Heuristic Research: Design, Methodology and Applications.* Newbury Park: Sage.

O'Hara, M. (1986) 'Heuristic inquiry as psychotherapy'. *Person-Centred Review,* 1 (2), 172–84.

Oakley, A. (1981) 'Interviewing women: a contradiction in terms' in Roberts, H. (ed.) *Doing Feminist Research.* London: Routledge.

Richards, A. (1974) 'Editor's Introduction' in Breuer, J. & Freud, S. *Studies on Hysteria.* Harmondsworth: Penguin.

Rogers, C. (1974) *On Becoming a Person.* London: Constable.

Rolfe, G. (1996) *Closing the Theory-Practice Gap: A New Paradigm for Nursing.* Oxford: Butterworth Heinemann.

Schön, D.A. (1983) *The Reflective Practitioner: How Professionals Think in Action.* London: Temple Smith.

Schön, D.A. (1987) *Educating the Reflective Practitioner.* San Francisco: Jossey-Bass.

Selltiz, C., Jahoda, M., Deutsch, M. & Cook, S.W. (1965) *Research Methods in Social Relations.* London: Methuen.

van Manen, M. (1997) *Researching Lived Experience.* 2nd edn. Ontario: The Althouse Press.

Index

Mezirow's model 74–5, 138, 139
Michaela (case example) 62–3
mid-life women 154–60
mirrors 6–7
Moustakas, C. 186–7
movement, creative 152–3, 154, 157, 158

narcissism 7
narrative
  autoethnography 30
  case example 130, 132–5
  concept 18
  critical care setting 40
  humanism 29
  nurse education 127
  philosophically congruent practice 35
  reflexive research process 75
  sharing 138
nature 156
needs, hierarchy 3
negative automatic thoughts 62
Newman's theory 149–52,
    153, 154, 155, 159
'nurse self' 30, 124
nurse–doctor interaction 47–9
nurse–patient relationships 123
nurse-artists 129–30
*Nursing Histories: Reviving life
  in abandoned selves* 165

objectivity 179–93
organismic self 2, 3, 4, 5

paradigms 17–18, 22–4
passive tense 181
paternalism 50
patterns 149, 154–60
personal boundaries 174–5
personal feelings 41–2
personal knowing 124
'personality' 10–11
perspectives, framing 44–54
Peter (student nurse) 95
philosophical aspects 22–35, 44, 45–7
poetry 85, 100, 107–18, 127, 130–1, 132
polemic 168
postmodern psychology 2, 60, 61
practitioner–client relationships 177
practitioners 6, 10–11, 17–20
praxis model 149–60

pregnancy, teenage 163, 166–9
problem framing 44, 52–3
professional boundaries 174–5
professional self 10–11, 88, 90, 94
professional socialisation 71, 72,
    89, 90, 93, 94, 95

rationality 189
'real' self *see* organismic self
reality perspective framing 44, 51–2
received concepts 9
reciprocity 122, 183, 184
reflection-in-action 125, 190, 191
reflection-on-action 65–76,
    114–15, 190
reflective practice 8, 28, 29
  caring self development 121–39
  critical care setting 39–54
  effectiveness measurement 53–4
  reality perspective framing 51–2
reflective research 188, 190
reflexivity 58–61, 65–76, 172, 179–93
relationships
  abusive 157–60
  caring 121–3
  practitioner–client 177
  researcher–researched
    180, 181, 182, 183, 184
relationships *cont.*
  teenage pregnancy 169
  to self, mid-life 156–7
rescuer, nurse as 172–4
research
  individual identity 162–77
  objectivity 162, 181
  perspective 145–94
  praxis model 149–60
  protocols disclosure 71, 72
  reflective 188, 190
  reflexive 65–76, 179–93
  self exploration 185–9
  use of self 182–4
  validity 191
researcher self 12–13, 76, 77
researcher/practitioner role 59, 61–79
respect for person 101
role framing 44, 47–50

scapegoats 147
science 162